Guided Self Meditations for Anxiety

Starts to Release Your Life from Anxiety and Stress Through Mindfulness Meditation, Self-Hypnosis and Spiritual Brain Healing to Relax, Deep Sleep and Be Happy.

Emily Write   Robert Peace

Anxiety is the space between 'now' and 'then'

Richard Abell

TABLE OF CONTENTS

INTRODUCTION

Anxiety or depression can make a person feel paralyzed over seemingly manageable situations. Do you ever think why you worry over things? Well, the reality is that the worry emanates from your mind other than the predicament or situation you are facing. The mind and body connection leads to physical impacts when one has an anxiety attack. Worrying causes fatigue, insomnia, muscle tension, irritability, twitching, digestive problems, and startled responses. While you might argue that the symptoms you experience are manageable, it is crucial to seek medical intervention and other non-intrusive relaxation approaches that will enable you to lead a healthy life. When you anticipate the worst in all situations, you might be unable to have healthy relationships, and your productivity dwindles. The condition makes people withdraw and treat their acquaintances with the utmost suspicion.

Anxiety can be an intense and overwhelming feeling. Be assured that you are not battling the condition alone. Millions of people worldwide suffer from an anxiety disorder. Notably, there is a difference between feeling anxious and clinical anxiety. The former can manifest through signs such as sweaty palms, chest tightness, stomach upsets, headaches, or heart palpitations. The occurrences result from the pumping of adrenaline. Anxiety as a disorder makes one experience excessive and persistent worry. In such instances, a person has no rational perspective and usually have unwarranted concerns. To manage anxiety, you will need a deep understanding of the condition.

Illustratively, an anxious mind equates to a room with thousands of drunken and unruly monkeys. The monkeys chatter endlessly and jump around without a care in the world. The highest voice of the clamoring monkeys is that of fear. This monkey is ever creating alarms in any slight situation. It creates thousands of 'what-if' scenarios, making anxious thoughts stay at our minds' forefronts. Fighting the monkeys can be tasking because they are an integral part of our consciousness. While we cannot banish these monkeys because they are part of us, we can tame them. Meditation allows you to listen and understand the chattering monkeys. Each meditation session familiarizes you with the good and bad behaviors of the monkey. You also get to understand their trigger points. Once you are the master, they learn to submit, and you can build a trusting and mutual relationship. Ultimately, you will enjoy calmness and happiness.

Meditation stops the perpetual chatter within our skulls. Thinking all the time can make one live in illusions. Meditation quiets an overactive mind. Learn to identify with the silence between all your mental actions. Meditation should be a regular practice that will help you realize that you are not your feelings or thoughts. The effectiveness of this practice is gradual, which makes it more sustainable than most medications. The detachment resulting from meditation allows you to rest in your being. Through meditation, you can address external triggers that threaten to disorient your inner peace. With intentionality, you can learn the meditation skills and use them at your convenient time or place. Whether you are on tranquilizers or any other medication that calms your nerves, meditation can be a complimentary practice you don't want to ignore.

CHAPTER 1: HOW TO CURE ANXIETY AND STRESS

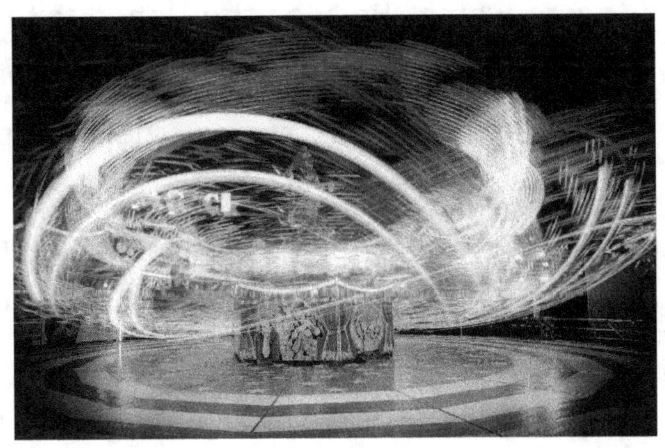

Anxiety is a natural response to fear or danger and can keep people safe in certain situations. Some people, however, experience anxiety more severely than others. This can lead to anxiety disorders, which can cause people to make major changes in their lives and habits to avoid situations or places that they believe cause them anxiety. If symptoms are persistent, a person might even be diagnosed with an anxiety disorder and recommended to seek treatment. Anxiety disorders can present themselves in a variety of ways; panic attacks, social anxiety, phobias, and separation anxiety to name a few.

A person might experience a host of physical symptoms with their anxiety, which can sometimes make it seem worse. Besides the unhealthy negative thoughts that are racing through their brain, they might also feel their heart racing, their temperature rising, or their breathing becoming shallower. These are all typical fight-or-flight responses that are triggered by anxiety to encourage a person to avoid the situation because the brain is perceiving it as a threat. It can be difficult for people to ignore thoughts of fear and dread when their body is pitching in and seemingly confirming them.

People experience anxiety for many different reasons, usually depending on their own life experiences and how their past has affected them. Some people have triggers for their anxiety, such as social situations or being separated from somewhere they feel is a safe space. Others feel anxiety in relation to nothing in particular but are constantly plagued with thoughts of fear and danger throughout the day. It can be difficult to deal with anxious feelings on a daily basis, but there are some things people can do to help ease the tension. This chapter discusses the psychology of anxiety, common symptoms, potential triggers, and ways to find relief.

Anxiety Explained

Anxiety can be difficult for people to recognize when they are first experiencing it. Most people, in fact, might mistake it for a physical health problem due to the symptoms that accompany it. At its core, anxiety is a response to stress. It makes people feel scared or worried about certain situations for a variety of reasons. Some people might be worried that others will judge them for how they act or speak, others might be afraid that some harm will come to them if they put themselves in a certain situation. These feelings are not all abnormal, however. Some common anxiety-inducing situations include a child's first day of school, an initial job interview, or someone's wedding day. These experiences can all cause anxiety due to the uncertainty of the situation and might cause a person to start thinking about worst-case scenarios.

All of these feelings are part of anxiety because it was the evolutionary way of keeping people safe when their environment was inherently dangerous. The heightening of senses and increased heart rate prepares the body to run or fight if presented with danger, which could have meant life or death in prehistoric times. Today, however, people are not faced with imminent death on a daily basis, but their brain might not know how to adjust itself to the safety of modern life. It can still trigger anxious feelings if it is threatened to encourage a person to flee the situation, even if the reasons are not rational.

Some people experience anxiety to an extreme degree and can feel like their negative thoughts are unrelenting. For someone with this level of anxiety, quieting their mind and finding any kind of relief can be especially difficult and might even seem impossible. If a person suffers from anxiety of this intensity for an extended period of time, they might fit the criteria for an anxiety disorder. Typically, to qualify for a disorder diagnosis, a person has to experience symptoms for longer than six months or the symptoms need to be interfering with their daily life.

There are a variety of anxiety disorders that are all defined by how the anxiety affects someone or what causes anxious feelings. Each person is different, even though they might experience similar symptoms of anxiety, and the way their anxiety affects them can make a big difference in a diagnosis. Among these disorders is a plethora of negative side effects caused by the increased levels of stress and constant negative thoughts. Some people have trouble sleeping at night, have trouble concentrating during the day, find interacting with others especially difficult, or are too afraid to leave their own homes.

Some common anxiety disorders include panic disorder, phobias, social anxiety disorder, and separation anxiety. Obsessive-compulsive disorder is no longer considered an anxiety disorder, but people diagnosed with it often experience severe anxiety as one of their symptoms. Each of these common disorders associate anxiety with a particular object, situation, or action. These disorders can severely affect a person's life by making them unable to perform daily tasks or prevent them from enjoying their hobbies. For example, someone with agoraphobia—fear of crowds—may become so debilitated by fear that they refuse to leave their home.

The symptoms of anxiety are not necessarily universal and can vary greatly from person to person. Sometimes the reason a person has anxiety can determine their symptoms, as well. For example, someone who has anxiety because they think they are in danger might feel a pounding heart because their body wants to escape. Another person, however, who is dreading a social interaction, might experience an upset stomach due to the increased stress. Symptoms can range from gastrointestinal issues to cardiovascular discomfort, headaches, and in extreme cases even vomiting if stress builds up enough with the anxiety.

At the onset of symptoms, some people may suddenly feel like they are no longer in control of their body. This can often increase feelings of anxiety because they may not feel like the dread or physical symptoms will ever subside. Sometimes this out of control feeling can even lead to panic attacks. Other startling symptoms can include nightmares or constantly recalling painful thoughts or memories.

These can also contribute to increased stress and anxiety because a person might feel like they cannot escape their own negative thoughts or what might seem to be an inevitably painful outcome of an event.

In people with generalized anxiety, it is more common to worry about things because of a past experience. For example, if a child's parent forgot them in a grocery store for an extended time, that child might then develop a fear of grocery stores and feel unsafe when they go to one. This could potentially carry on into adulthood, even if the person doesn't remember the event that instigated their anxiety. Common symptoms of this type of anxiety usually present themselves when a person is in a certain situation or sometimes if they merely consider putting themselves in the trigger situation. These people often experience a racing heart, shortness of breath or rapid breathing, restlessness, trouble focusing, and a slew of other symptoms.

Anxiety can even affect a person's stomach function, causing gas, constipation, or diarrhea when it flares up. This can also contribute to more severe anxiety in a person because they may become fixated on their stomach problems and convinced that if they are in a social situation, they might have a problem they cannot get away to handle. Some people can experience this discomfort even at the thought of doing something that gives them anxiety. This is why it can be particularly difficult for people to overcome their anxiety. If even the thought of doing something makes them feel physically ill, it can be difficult to convince themselves that actually doing it won't be painful.

When people experience these intense physical symptoms in relation to their anxiety, it can often cause them to start avoiding things, situations, or people that they believe will trigger their negative feelings. Although this might seem like an effective coping mechanism to those with anxiety, it can actually severely limit their lives by making them unable to participate in normal everyday tasks. On top of wanting to avoid these situations, anxiety can make a person feel too weak or fatigued to engage in social activities. This further cements their desire to withdraw and stay confined to their safe space instead of facing and managing their anxiety.

Causes and treatments

Most people feel anxious at some point in their life, but there can be certain factors or triggers that cause other people to feel it more severely than normal. These can include someone's genetics, their environment, how their brain is wired, and what life experiences they've had. If a person associates something with fear, it is likely they will develop anxiety surrounding that thing. Although it is typical for people to have some sort of trigger for their anxiety, this is not true for all cases. Some people have very generalized anxiety about nothing in particular; they are simply always worried or dreading being out in the world.

For some people, one type of anxiety can cause them to develop another type of anxiety. For example, someone who has anxiety about suffering harm or getting sick might develop a germ-related obsessive-compulsive disorder as a way to ensure they will never get sick. Or, people with social anxiety disorder might eventually develop agoraphobia if they never force themselves to interact with others.

Risk factors for different types of anxiety disorders typically coexist in people who suffer with them, which demonstrates that no single experience is likely to cause someone to develop a disorder. Scientists have found that nature and nurture are strongly linked when it comes to the likelihood that someone will develop severe anxiety. Genetically, research has shown that people have about a 30 to 67 percent chance of inheriting anxiety from their parents (Carter, n.d.). Although someone's DNA might be a factor in them developing anxiety, it cannot account for all of the reasons that have developed it.

Environmental factors should also be taken into consideration when trying to find the root cause of anxiety. Parenting style can be a large factor in whether or not a person will develop anxiety. If parents are controlling of their children or if they model anxious behaviors, the child might grow up thinking these are normal behaviors they should model. This can lead to feeling anxious based on a learned behavior. Other factors such as continual stress, abuse, or loss of a loved one can also elicit a severe anxious reaction because a person may not know how to handle the situation they find themselves in.

In addition to the environment, a person's health can often cause anxiety as well. If someone is diagnosed or living with a chronic medical condition or a severe illness, it can cause an anxious reaction. One possibility is if the illness is affecting the person's hormones which can cause stress, or if their feelings of not having control are worsened by a diagnosis they cannot fix.

Some people might not realize that the choices they make daily could be contributing to their anxiety. Things such as excessive caffeine, tobacco use, and not exercising enough can all cause anxiety. Caffeine and other stimulants can increase a person's heart rate and simulate anxiety symptoms. Not exercising can lower a person's level of happy hormones and make their muscles tense or sore which can also contribute to stress. A person's personality can also determine how severe their anxiety might be. Shy people who tend to stay away from conversations and interaction might develop more severe social anxiety because they are not exposed to those situations often.

When experiencing anxiety, it can seem like there is no way out, but there are actually quite a few different ways a person can work to ease their worries, ranging from clinical to holistic approaches. What type of treatments will work depends on the person, and often, how severe their struggle is.

A few clinical ways to treat anxiety include counseling, psychotherapy, and medication. These are not the only ways a person can be medically treated, but they tend to be the most conventional routes for treating mental illness. Counseling is a type of therapy where the person is able to talk to a licensed practitioner and receive feedback and advice about their situation and how to handle their emotions. Most counselors have a master's degree in the psychology field and are licensed through their state. This type of therapy is usually considered a short-term solution for people who are struggling but not debilitated by their anxiety.

Psychotherapy is typically a more long-term solution for people whose lives are impacted by their anxiety. This type of therapy can focus on a broader range of issues and triggers such as a person's anxious patterns or behaviors and how to fix them. Cognitive behavioral therapy is often used in this type of therapy to work with the person to adjust their thoughts and behaviors.

Some people find relief once prescribed medication to help them manage their anxiety. This route is usually reserved for people who are struggling the most and having trouble calming themselves on their own. There are various types of medications such as SSRIs (selective serotonin reuptake inhibitors) and SNRIs (serotonin-norepinephrine reuptake inhibitors) that alter brain chemicals to reduce anxiety or worry.

Making changes to their lifestyle and habits can also help people with anxiety relieve some of their symptoms. This is a more natural approach to managing anxiety and can be successful for people who are dedicated to making positive life changes. Small things such as diet adjustments and increasing activity levels can reduce anxious feelings. Establishing a consistent sleep schedule is also important to help someone ensure they are getting enough rest each night. Stress fatigues the body and it may need more time to fully recuperate at night if it was taxed during the day. Making sure the body has a routine can also make someone feel safe and know what to expect from their day.

Meditation can also be a good way for people to calm their minds and ease anxiety. Taking time during the day to be still and quiet might help someone stop the constant worry they feel during the day and relax for a moment. Once they start training their body to relax, it is more likely that they can keep it up during the day. Finally, avoiding stimulants such as caffeine, sugar, and tobacco, and depressants such as alcohol can greatly improve a person's chances of overcoming their anxiety. These substances contribute to the brain's hyperactivity and can often increase feelings of anxiety.

Recognizing Stress: How to Calm your Body

Did you know that one-third of the United States population reported to experiencing extreme levels of stress? These statistics was obtained from a 2007 poll of the American Psychological Association. This was more than a decade ago. Now imagine what the percentage will be now with all that's going on in the free world. Stress has the tendency of making people feel overwhelmed with the goings-on around them. According to that poll, about one in every five persons reported that they experience high levels of stress not less than fifteen days in every month. Although it has been proved that low levels of stress do not pose any immediate threat to your health, but escalated and poorly managed stress can produce life threatening conditions. Your ability to recognize high stress levels and the stressors will help you know the exact ways to act promptly in the healthiest ways that will help you change unhealthy behaviors thereby regaining and maintaining control over your health. And for you to achieve this there are situations you must pay attention. Paying attention to those situations will help you understand your stress pattern, the stressors, and how you can avoid future occurrence.

You should be aware of your stress pattern

Being that everyone experiences stress differently and on different occasions, understanding how your stress occurs, what your stressors are and how you get to understand that you are stressed will go a long way in helping you maintaining calmness during and after a stressful episode. Also, your ability to understand how you react to stressful situations is also important. This concerns your thoughts and behavior and how they align with or react to your stressors and stress. When you understand this, you will be able to point out the difference in your behavior during the times you are stressed and the times when you're not.

You should identify the sources of your stress

Identifying the sources of your stress also means shooting the dart on your stressors. To do this effectively, you have to be more attentive to the moments before a stressful situation. The reason for the extra attention is for you to identify the particular events or situations that trigger stress feelings. Being able to do this will go a long way in helping you plan your life or change your lifestyle. For instance, if you discover that the relationship that exists between you and your family members, or between you and your employer or a colleague at work, or the relationship that exists between you and a neighbor is your stressor, what you do after this discovery will determine whether you deal with stress and maintain good health, or whether these stressors will continue to haunt you at the expense of your health.

There is also the possibility of your stressor arising from financial predicaments or decisions. It could be from much workload or the lack of a job. It could be from the consequences of a bad decision. Whatever you identify as your stressor, you should know that taking steps to avoid or discontinue their activities in your life will help you calm your body.

You should be aware of your own stress signal

Not everybody experiences the same signs and symptoms of stress. Whereas some people's manifestation might show minor signs like increased heartbeat and profuse sweating, some other people's manifestation might be observed through major signs like heightened alertness, extreme anxiety or panic attacks. You might realize that when you are stressed, you usually have a hard time articulating your thoughts well or failing at general body coordination. But this might be for you and your way of showing signs of stress. For someone else, it may be inability to concentrate, inability or difficulty in making sound decision, anger and rage mostly over minor issues, headaches and migraine, muscle tension or excessive tiredness. Amongst all these signals and the ones not mentioned, knowing what your signal is will help you identify stressful moments. This way you will be better informed on how to handle them and calm your body at the same time.

You should identify how you deal with stress

How do you deal with stress? Do you calm yourself by engaging in healthy activities or do you worsen your situation by practicing unhealthy behaviors like drinking, smoking, taking hard drugs, engaging in sexual adventures, denying yourself food, binge eating, or all of them? If the way you deal with stress is by engaging in the above bad habits, then you should know that the relief you think you get from them is just temporal. Such activities will not help you calm your body, and if you do them as often as you're stressed, you will develop an addiction to them. You already know how burdensome and unhealthy addictive behaviors are; you should have the presence of mind to avoid them. There are healthy ways to deal with stress and these ways will be explained in as the book progresses.

Being able to identify these behaviors as coping mechanism will help you understand how your body reacts to stress and what you should do to restore calmness to your body.

Identifying healthy ways to manage your stress

There are tons of stress-reducing and controlling activities you can engage in, if you want to effectively manage your stress and emerge from it healthier and renewed. You should consider all the stress management tips available such as meditation, exercising, therapies (with include talking to a professional psychologist, attending group interactive sessions, taking up cognitive behavior therapy sessions, talking to families, friends and other people you feel safe to talk to, and seeing a life coach), and engaging in activities that calms your mind.

Your ability to identify healthy ways to deal with stress should also include avoiding every form of unhealthy behavior. You should keep it in mind that unhealthy behaviors develop gradually, and when they are learned you find them a tad bit difficult to unlearn. Hence, in learning new and rewarding behaviors and habits and dropping negative ones, you should follow a gradual process. If you try to drop them all at once, it might prove much of a task for you. Remember that the target is to enter and remain in a state of calmness.

Learn how to care for yourself

There is no perfect way to care for yourself, but there is always the right way to care for yourself. If you discover that a certain behavior is inimical to your wellbeing, you should drop it. Several ways abound how you can care for yourself in the healthiest way, and they include:

- Maintaining a healthy diet.

- Ensuring you have adequate sleep.

- Drinking the recommended five liters of water.

- Engaging in regular physical and mental exercises. These include all the physical exercises according to the recommendation of your health care provider and other mind exercises like yoga and mindfulness meditation.

Always make yourself available to be helped or supported

In whatever that concerns behavioral abnormality, seeking help is always the key. Sometimes people who are facing a lot of things do think they are the only ones going through that phase. But the moment you open up to people and tap into the help they have to offer; you will realize that you are not alone in your world. Accepting help from the people who matter in your life will go a long way to help you deal with stress and stressful situations. It will also help you understand how best to avoid stressful situations, and most importantly, you will learn how to calm your body. The knowledge in the minds of everyone is deep, and it might interest you that the problem which you previously held as unsolvable is actually solvable if you reach out to people, let them know how you feel, and allow them teach you a thing or two about practical ways to manage stress through doing all the things that will help you calm your body.

CHAPTER 2: POSITIVE THINKING & POSITIVE AFFIRMATIONS

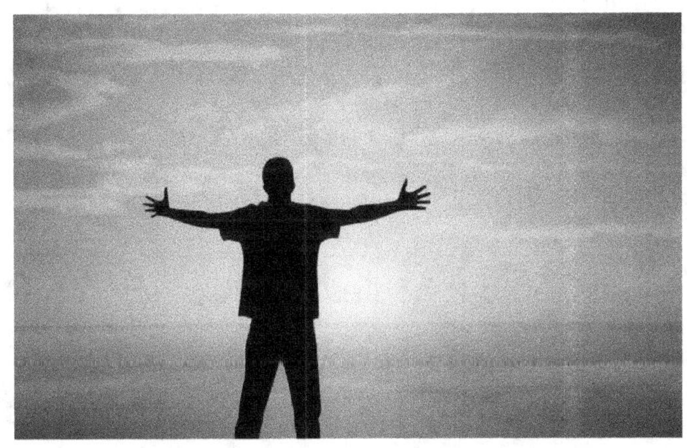

Positive Thinking Can Assist Healing

Recognizing that you have the power within you to believe anything and everything is possible is a very good beginning and a positive way to get your mind and body ready for the journey of healing.

When you have faith and really believe in the work that you are doing, positive outcomes are usually in the future for you. If you continue to eat well and practice different types of meditation while being mindful and positive, you will have more confidence and a level of belief that is powerful and that power can be tapped into.

And it is not just believing in the things that you are doing, but it is also welcoming challenges and changes and being open to all kinds of different possibilities! Holding onto that deep belief that anything can change at any time for the better.

Our minds and our bodies already work together as an all-star team, even when we are not aware of it, so why not add positivity to that operation!! It is going on whether we participate or not, so just remember to insert as many positive affirmations and new beliefs as possible into your mind on a daily basis.

It is the same as when you have an old house, and you start to fix it up and remodel it. You begin to add new paint, you put in new floors, new carpet, new walls and then brand new ceilings.

You can do the same thing with your mind, body, and spirit by being positive and adding new, bright, important, motivating positive and inspiring things into them daily. Your system will start to believe all of those positive and beautiful things that are being fed into it, and this will assist in your healing. We are also able to take advantage of the power of our minds to manipulate our immune systems in order to lower our risk of getting injuries or diseases.

This chapter is focused on being completely positive and putting positivity into your mind and spirit. You should, from this day forward, make a choice to feel good rather than allowing outside elements to control the way that you feel.

This will not be easy, especially if you are only used to getting negative vibrations from everyone, including yourself, but you will be able to achieve it with much dedication and practice.

You see, positive thinking is not about fooling yourself; it is more about changing the way you see things and beginning to look at a different side of reality. Once again, it is the ability to reframe any situation and see the positive when you have convinced yourself that there is only negativity present.

Positive thoughts and affirmations deposits are just another way to help in the important process of developing self-love, recognizing your self-worth, and getting deeper in touch with your true self.

When you are happy and positive, you promote positivity and happiness. You are very calm, and you have very effective communication with other people. When you place value on positive thoughts and healthy living, others can tell because it's all in your energy. The best way to reframe something is by using humor.

Having a positive outlook can mean the difference between succeeding and failing or even being happy and being miserable. But if you try to maintain an outlook that is positive, your life will change for the better. You will be happier, healthier, and more peaceful.

The only thing that separates a winner from a loser is that when a winner fails, they will start over and try again, but when a loser fails, they will just simply give up and quit.

The more you expect to be successful, the more success you will achieve. The more you see a positive outcome, the more your mind and focus will be on making sure that happens. You deserve greatness, so expect nothing less than that for yourself, your life, and your future.

Having a positive attitude can make a bad situation turn better, and it can also make you happier, healthier, and more productive. Most importantly, it can bring you true success by allowing you to live in peace and truth with yourself.

This is just another tip to keep inserting positive thoughts to replace negative ones. If your pants are old and from the thrift store, then focus on that nice shirt you are wearing, because there is always something more positive that you can think about.

Stop Waiting For Someone Else To Change You!! Most of these quick-fix schemes, self-help DVD's or books will not do you any good unless you make the decision and demonstrate the commitment to change within yourself.

Surround yourself with positive thinkers and people who think you are great, and they will show you by example, the amount of difficulties that need to be faced in order to create change. These individuals will have a true understanding, commitment, and desire to keep themselves motivated.

Positive thoughts are always a good way to start your day, along with your morning stretches. Remember each day to recognize your power, claim it, and plan on how you are going to use it at that particular time. Choosing positive self-messages, adjusting your attitude, automatically thinking from a gratitude perspective and celebrating your strength, all of this should prepare you to have a great day.

Delete It

I want you to make a trash bin so that you can throw away all of those negative emotions, memories, and thoughts. You are going to start dumping plenty of negative feelings and emotions into this trash can, and it will feel great while doing so!! If you have a bad day and you are not feeling motivated or inspired, write down how you feel and place it into your trash bin.

All of those feelings, thoughts, and emotions that you have been holding inside will go into this box because you are no longer holding anything inside! This will be extremely useful if you have suffered childhood trauma of any kind and have been holding onto it ever since.

Write down exactly what happened to you word for word, do not leave anything out at all, and when you have finished, place it into this box. Anything negative or bad that you may have survived, write it down and throw it in here as well, because you are going to be releasing all of those memories from your spirit so you can refresh and recharge. You are to be very honest and write down exactly what happened and how it made you feel.

Love Yourself Through Setbacks

Life happens, things take the wrong types of terms; we make mistakes, and situations don't work out the way they're supposed to. When you run into a difficult or a stressful situation or even a very painful one like the loss of a family member or a loved one, it really helps to be self-compassionate and patient with yourself and learn how to love yourself through all your failures and setbacks.

Life and setbacks are going to be hard enough to deal with. The last thing you need to be doing is putting more pressure on yourself and add it to your stress by being judgmental and critical.

When you learn to really love yourself and understand yourself and forgive yourself through these types of times, it makes you eliminate a lot of anger and depression when you have to deal with pain and horrible experiences.

The negative emotional reactions that you have to life situations should be very minimal. You should be able to accept responsibility for a negative event but don't feel negative about it.

Do not judge yourself about a negative outcome or failed marriage or relationship or job. Just look at yourself with kindness, forgive yourself, be compassionate, and stay grounded and focused. Because, guess what, you are going to continue to move forward in life and be just fine.

The power of the human spirit is filled with so many possibilities within ourselves that we can do whatever we dream and desire and we shouldn't have to settle for mediocre lives.

We can be ambitious and dream and never give up and constantly strive to achieve the things we want. It is well worth the time, energy, and hard work that will be invested to see success and happiness, a true fulfillment at the end of achieving your goals.

There is a strong and close relationship between pursuing challenging goals and being truly happy and fulfilled. Truly happy people live an optimistic type of life because they believe in their capabilities and in their dreams, and they believe in each step that they take to achieve their goals. Most people who live a peaceful and happy life know that they have a purpose, and they are either living it or trying to find it.

It has stated in studies that happy people live longer, they have more friends, they are healthier, and that is because they have a positive outlook on life and they are always working towards something.

CHAPTER 3: MEDITATION TECHNIQUES AND ROUTINE AND HOW TO MEDITATE

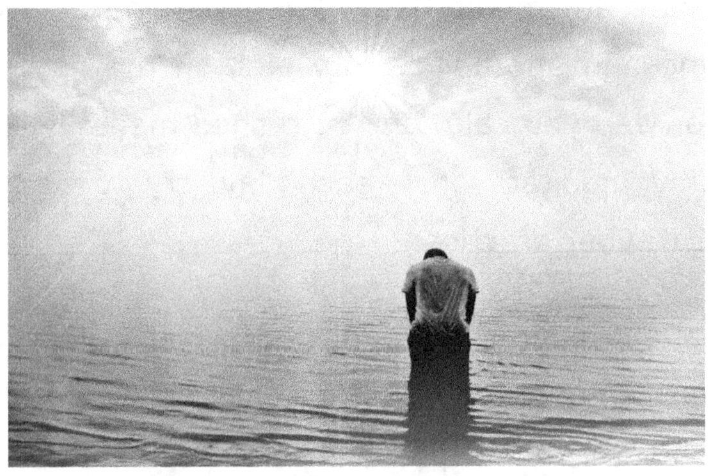

As you've seen, meditation can be practiced anywhere. Usually, it helps to be alone. However, many larger cities have meditation centers, where you can go and meditate in a room with others. The atmosphere will be quiet and conducive to a peaceful visit.

An open church is an ideal spot, as well, by peaceful methods. Silent mantra meditation works nicely in a quiet, spiritual atmosphere. Christian churches often have stained glass windows, which are ideal for visual methods. The colors and picture will slowly draw you in, leaving your thoughtful comments behind.

Many meditators try to spend two short periods each day in meditation. Twenty minutes in the morning and another twenty later in the day works well to keep you calm and refreshed mentally. If you can only meditate once each day, try to add a bit longer to your practice.

To avoid being disturbed, find a place alone. Turn off your cell phone and put it out of sight so that you won't be worried. If possible, dim the lights. Finally, close the door to keep pets away. Just as they curl up in your lap when you rest or nap, they will sense your calm mind and try to be near you. A happy dog in your lap does not lead to successful meditation.

Advice

Meditation, unlike hypnosis and other states of altered consciousness, has no suspected dangers. You can't get "stuck" in a meditative state, and no one has control over your thoughts or actions. So you have nothing to fear from trying it out. What you have to gain is less tension, lower blood pressure, and control over life's stress.

To begin exploring meditation, try out the methods described here. See which ones fit your life best. See which ones work better and relax you more. The truth is that all of the research into meditation won't affect you. What will make a difference is how the practice makes a difference in your life. To help evaluate, make yourself a little checklist:

Do I feel relaxed and calm after meditating?

Are there any unpleasant results? (Groggy, Tired)

Did any methods seem to work best?

Did any methods seem not to work as well?

Will I try meditating again tomorrow?

What does it feel like when you meditate? But as you progress, you may feel a sense of sinking slowly, hearing noises as though you're in a peaceful tunnel. If an alarm or phone rings, you'll be pulled back "up" to full alertness at once. You may feel dizzy if it happens. To avoid this happening too frequently, turn off or silence your cell phone before beginning to meditate. You probably will feel a little dizzy when you "come back" from meditating. You've been losing less oxygen and your pulse is slowed, so give yourself a moment or two to adjust, when you stop.

Honestly, any time you introduce a new habit or practice that will change how you feel, how you react to stress, and how your body responds to tension, it's a a significant change. Life lets us get conditioned. So to change sometimes, we need to do a little re-conditioning. Try the techniques that work best for several days at least. See how you feel in a few days as opposed to after one try. If you feel adventurous, try another technique or combine a couple. The only result can be the improvement. The less we let stress and tension affect us, the healthier and happier we will be.

How to Meditate

Meditation is a great - and logically demonstrated - habit for a solid body and mind. Be that as it may, a few people battle with the time, consistency, center and system required to get meditation right.

What a great many people don't know is, you don't really need to take a seat and close your eyes for a considerable length of time a day - in light of the fact that there are other far less demanding approaches to get your psyche into a thoughtful state, and appreciate the advantages of this ancient practice.

For example:

1. While you walk your dog

As you're strolling Jack, instead of meditating a large number of things you're stalling on, take a stab at giving careful attention to your environment.

Recognize the sounds, the general population, the climate. What do you smell? What would you be able to see? What would you be able to hear out yonder? How does your body feel?

By taking a careful walk, you're discharging endorphins, which enable you to build your joy level, and even diminish stress and live longer.

2. While you make coffee or tea

- Begin your morning with more profound concentration, lucidity and peace by rehearsing this simple reflective custom.

As you make your tea or coffee, concentrate your attention on your developments.

- Close your eyes and notice the tea, take a taste, enjoy it. Furthermore, as you experience the ritual custom, be deliberately mindful of your breath.
- You can likewise apply this while you cook your most loved supper or heat.
- 3. While you do the dishes
- Doing dishes or clearing your floor doesn't need to be an errand. Actually, this is the ideal time for you to associate with yourself and feel grounded.
- Concentrate on your breath, and your body's sensations.
- On the off chance that you see your mind wandering, take yourself back to mindfulness by thinking about the general

population and things throughout your life that fill you with delight and appreciation.

4. While you shower

- Have you at any point asked why your best thoughts tend to come while you're showering?

- "The shower is where we can develop mindfulness. When we get tranquil, when we get still, when we rest, you could state, in mindfulness, our natural drive to see associations that we didn't see the prior minute is unobstructed."

- On the off chance that you need to take it somewhat further, as you shower, you can even envision accomplishing your objectives, and the feeling that will wash over you as you do.

5. While you tune in to your main tune

- Practicing mindfulness or meditation can be as straightforward as tuning in to your main song - insofar as you're totally centered around your breathing and the feeling that the song brings out in you.

6. While you ride the transport or sit in your auto

- Sit serenely. Take long and full breaths. Recognize the warm sun stroking your face. Welcome the delightful city lights or scene. Also, let your mind take you all alone trip.

As you now know, the benefits of meditation can be conveyed into the most ordinary exercises - helping you acknowledge life all the more, inhabit a slower pace, embrace new propensities, and be more joyful.

Practical Advice on meditation

- To what extent Should I Meditate?

In the event that you are new to meditation, I suggest beginning gradually. Begin with only 5 minutes every day. Bit by bit increment the time more than half a month. When I began reflecting, five minutes felt like an unfathomable length of time. I now practice for 30 minutes every day, and here and there I am astonished at how rapidly it passes!

Where Should I Meditate?

Locate an comfortable spot where you can sit. You can sit on the floor (utilizing a pad or pad for help if necessary) or sit upright in a seat, with your feet laying on the floor.

A few people suggest that you don't rests on your back, however I figure you ought to think in whatever stance works for you (unless resting influences you to fall asleep!)

You can meditate anyplace, yet I like having an extraordinary place in my home for my training. You can take in more about making a meditation space in your home here.

What Do I Do?

The least demanding meditation strategy is to count the breath. I forget about each in-breath and breath with a similar number. So, my mind concentrates on "One" (in-breath), "One" (out-breath), "Two" (in-breath), "Two" (out-breath), et cetera. When I hit 10 (which seldom occurs before my mind has wandered!) I begin once again at one. On the off chance that you don't care for counting, you can essentially rehash to yourself "in, out…. in, out… "

At the point when your mind wanders, which it WILL DO (that's what the mind does!) tenderly guide your attention back to your breath. On the off chance that you have to begin once again counting in light of the fact that you don't recollect the latest relevant point of interest, that is fine! The key is to not reprimand or judge yourself for giving your attention a chance to wander. Actually …

seeing that your psyche has wandered is the general purpose of meditation you are winding up more mindful of the activities of your mind!

Indeed, even the moderately basic guideline to "take after the breath" can sound somewhat obscure or confounding. A supportive method is to bring your attention where you most notice the vibe of the breath — in the chest and lungs? the nose? the stomach? That is your stay. Each time your mind wanders, return to the physical vibes of relaxing.

At the point when thought emerge, it's anything but difficult to get diverted and tail them and draw in them and explain them and investigate them… . An accommodating practice is to just name the contemplations: "stressing," "arranging," "recollecting." Don't stress over making sense of the exact mark for the kind of thought you're having. Simply "considering" will do, as well!

- What's more, if the thoughts don't leave? It's still alright.
- I adore that depiction of the training.

How Do I Fit This Into My Day?

The critical thing is to make it a propensity. After numerous long stretches of a reliable practice, it will end up being a vital piece of your day, such as practicing or brushing your teeth!

Changing your habits over some stretch of time really makes new neural systems in your mind, and the training will turn out to be a piece of your day by day schedule.

Knocks along the Road

- In any case, Nothing's Happening!

Meditation is about non-judgmental mindfulness. We have to not bring desires into our practice. You may encounter a snapshot of significant understanding amid a meditation session. Or, then again you may be truly exhausted. You may feel fretful and disturbed. Or, on the other hand you may feel quiet and relaxed.

Meditation is tied in with grasping whatever is right now. The advantages of meditation — more noteworthy mindfulness and discretion, increased calm and empathy — will rise after some time. In any case, every individual session will be totally unique.

So, in case you're exhausted, simply take note of, "This is the thing that fatigue feels like." If you're content, take note of, "This is the thing that satisfaction feels like."

•Meditating for 10 minutes daily is limitlessly superior to meditating for 70 minutes once per week. Attempt to meditate oftentimes (consistently if conceivable), regardless of the possibility that that just means sitting for a couple of minutes.

•Start little. In the event that you endeavor to meditate for 30 minutes right from the beginning, I can practically ensure that you will get disappointed and disheartened. I prescribe beginning with five minutes, and just increase that time when you're comfortable. Regardless of the possibility that you sit for five minutes, and you find that your mind wanders the entire time, you will in any case get unfathomable advantages from meditation.

•Pick a gentle alarm. On the off chance that your clock is uproarious and jolting, reckoning the caution will occupy your attention amid meditation.

•Meditate in a peaceful place. Having less distractions around you will normally enable you to meditate better, and will make your meditation significantly more profitable.

•Its most straightforward to lose your attention amid your out-breath. You're in-breath is exceptionally articulated and simple to focus on, and the vast majority's mind wanders on their out-breaths (me included). These merits remembering.

•Be simple on yourself when your mind wanders. It's

anything but difficult to wind up plainly disappointed with yourself when your mind wanders, yet don't. Your meditations will be substantially more gainful when you delicately bring your mind back.

CHAPTER 4: A BREATHING TECHNIQUE TO HELP COMBAT INSOMNIA

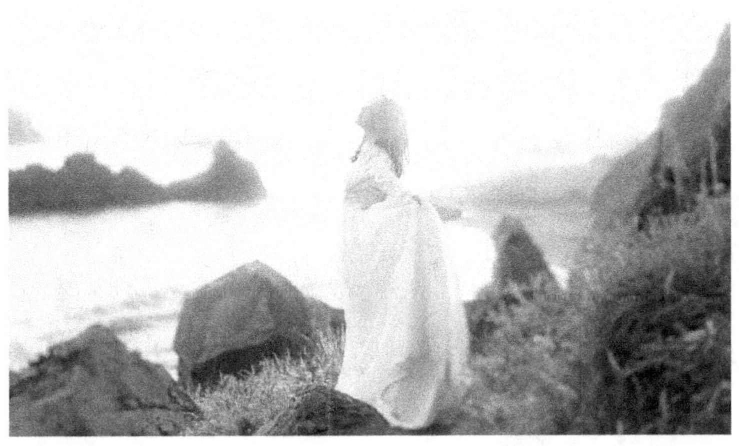

There is an assortment of relaxation techniques systems to look over. Successful completion of relaxation techniques for longer time provides benefits which help us in increasing level of productivity and ability to relax, including the improvement of a positive energy. The benefits are multifold-reduced muscle tension, along these lines, lessening the body's requirement for oxygen and decreasing exhaustion and uneasiness.

Focus on Breathing

If you find that stress is causing you to lose your sleep, this relaxation technique can be sought. Focusing on breath, would help you to relax your mind and reduce worries and stress. Since deep breathes infuse more oxygen in your bloodstream, profound breathing helps you unwind. If you are doing it for the first time, there could be some difficulty but eventually your body will get used to it.

To enable yourself to concentrate on your breathing, it is better to find a solitary, empty space. Dim light conditions are preferable as they help soothe our mood. This isn't at all mandatory to follow this rule; however, it can enable you to concentrate on the training in case you are amateurs.

Locate an agreeable, calm spot to sit or rest

Take your place

Sit straight and relaxed

Take a moment to get comfortable

Don't do anything

Just sit completely relaxed for a few minutes

Make sure there is nothing disturbing you

Now, close your eyes

Then put your one hand on our lower midsection

Breath normally

Keep your focus on your breathing

Inhale, and watch the air travel through your body

Exhale and let the air take away all your thoughts and negativity

Inhale

Exhale

Take a long slow, deep breath in

And slowly exhale

Attempt to take a whole breath so your lungs are full

Feel the air coming in through your nose move descending, extending your lungs completely and your lower midsection rises

Inhale out through your mouth

And exhale

Repeat few times more

You are becoming very relaxed

Breathe out

Release all tension and stress

Breathe in

With each breath the air infuses calmness

Breathe out

Feel the air leaving your body conveys strain, worries and stress with it

Now put one hand just underneath our belly button

Loosen up your stomach muscles

Inhale

Exhale

As you continue with the deep breathing

Feel your hand rise a little (and fall as you exhale)

Inhale

Exhale

Your chest rises marginally, as well, working together with your midriff

Inhale

Exhale

As you breathe out gradually, it would be more relaxing to allow any sound made by your throat come out

You must not hold back

Use the chanting word would "Om" to help you

Utter these words as you exhale

Take a deep breath in

Now exhale: "Oooooommm"

Again, take a deep breath in

And exhale: "Oooooommm"

If any distracting thought occurs

Don't worry about it, it may happen

Use the "Oooooommm" word to find your focus

Take a deep breath in

Now exhale: "Oooooommm"

Again, take a deep breath in

And exhale: "Oooooommm"

Now start breathing normally

Stabilize your breathing

Let it return to its normal rate

Remain seated with your eyes closed

Try to feel your surrounding

You are feeling completely relaxed now

There is no worries, anxiety, or stress

You are very calm

You can open your eyes.

Deep Breathing

Deep breathing is a simple method to unwind and release your stresses. Likewise called belly breathing, diaphragmatic breathing, and stomach breathing, it can bring down your pulse and loosen up tense muscles. It can enable you to wash away a portion of the worry of your day and get ready for a more settled, more loosening up night. Pick a period that works for you. Attempt to keep a similar everyday practice once a day to pick up the most advantage out of it.

You can do it essentially anyplace, and it just takes a couple of minutes. In case you're fatigued and don't have 10 minutes to de-stress, even a couple of full breaths can help. When you've drilled it a couple of times, a small-scale variant of this activity can help ease stress. Simply envision that every breath is clearing ceaselessly pressure, and you may quiet your uneasiness in one moment or two.

When you figure out how to profound inhale, you can utilize it to quiet you anyplace. When you're sitting at your work area or doing work around the house, know about your breathing and the pressure you are feeling. Keep in mind your profound breathing everyday practice and let the pressure blur away. Utilize this bit by bit manual for figure out how to overwhelm your stress.

Locate an agreeable, calm spot to sit or rests

Pick a spot where you realize you won't be aggravated

Take your place

Stay calm and relaxed

Take a moment to get comfortable

Don't do anything

Just stay completely relaxed for a few minutes

Make sure there is nothing disturbing you

Notice if there is tension anywhere

If you feel any part tense, release the tension

Adjust your body to release the pressure

On the off chance that sitting, keep your back straight and your feet level on the floor

Now, close your eyes

Start by breathing normally

Inhale

Exhale

Don't try to increase or decrease the rate of your breathing

Just focus on your breathing

Inhale

Exhale

Put one hand on your midsection, just underneath your ribs

Focus as the hand on your midsection goes in with the breath

Take a deep breath through your nose

1...2...3...4

Make sure your chest does not rise while your stomach expands

Holding your breath

Breathe out through your mouth

4...3...2...1

Do this practice multiple times until you have a quieting beat

Inhale gradually through your nose

1...2...3...4

Holding your breath

Gradually exhale through your mouth

4...3...2...1

Inhale

As you breathe in, envision that the air you're breathing is spreading unwinding sensation all through your body

Holding your breath

Exhale

As you breathe out, envision that your breath is whooshing ceaselessly stress and strain

Repeat this process a few more times

Breathe in

1...2...3...4

Hold your breath in the abdomen

Exhale through your mouth

4...3...2...1

Breathe in

Every inhaling is energizing

Hold your breath

Exhale through your mouth

Every exhaling is calming and relaxing

Breathe in

1...2...3...4

Hold your breath in the abdomen

Exhale through your mouth

4...3...2...1

Breathe in

1...2...3...4

Hold your breath in the abdomen

Exhale through your mouth

4...3...2...1

Now stabilize your breath

Feel how relaxed you are

All the stress was released

Your mind is calm and clear

You are in a perfect harmony

Take this feeling with you

Now open your eyes.

Roll Breathing

Roll breathing causes you to grow full utilization of your lungs and to concentrate on your relaxing. You can do it in any position. Yet, while you are learning, it is ideal to lie on your back with your knees bowed.

Practice move breathing day by day for a little while until you can do it anyplace. You can utilize it as a moment unwinding apparatus whenever you need one. Some individuals get tipsy the initial couple of times they attempt move relaxing. In the event that you start to inhale excessively quick or feel woozy, slow your relaxing. Get up gradually.

Locate an agreeable, calm spot to sit or rests

Pick a spot where you realize you won't be aggravated

Lie on your back

Bow your knees

Stay calm and relaxed

Take a moment to get comfortable

Don't do anything

Just stay completely relaxed for a few minutes

Make sure there is nothing disturbing you

Notice if there is tension anywhere

If you feel any part tense, release the tension

Adjust your body to release the pressure

Now, close your eyes

Start by breathing normally

Inhale

Exhale

Do not rush the process

Just focus on your breathing

Inhale

Exhale

1

Put your left hand on your tummy and your right hand on your chest

Notice how your hands move as you are breathing in and out

2

Work on filling your belly by breathing so that your left hand goes up when you breathe in and your right hand on the chest stays still

Continuously take in through your nose

Now add the second means to your breathing

Breathe in first into your belly as in the past

And after that keep breathing in into your upper chest

3

Inhale gradually and routinely

As you do as such

Your right hand will rise

And your left hand will fall a little as your tummy falls

4

Now inhale out the air first from your belly

And only then from your chest

Notice how at first your left hand

And afterward your right hand fall

As you breathe out gradually through your mouth

Make calm, whooshing sound
Repeat these 6 to 8 times

Inhale gradually with your belly

Then inhale slowly with your chest

Now exhale gradually with your belly

Then exhale slowly with your chest

Notice that the development of your belly and chest rises and falls

Like the movement of moving waves

As you breathe in,

Notice the energy flowing your body

As you become full of vitality

As you breathe out

Feel the strain leaving your body

As you become increasingly loose

Inhale gradually with your belly

Then inhale slowly with your chest

Now exhale gradually with your belly

Then exhale slowly with your chest

Inhale gradually with your belly

Then inhale slowly with your chest

Now exhale gradually with your belly

Then exhale slowly with your chest

Inhale gradually with your belly

Then inhale slowly with your chest

Now exhale gradually with your belly

Then exhale slowly with your chest

Inhale gradually with your belly

Then inhale slowly with your chest

Now exhale gradually with your belly

Then exhale slowly with your chest

Now bring your breathing back to normal

Remain lying for a while

Became aware of everything in and around you

Now open your eyes.

Box Breathing

One of the simplest and best breath work procedures is box breathing. No, this doesn't include sitting in one of those goliath boxes you get when you move to another house, yet rather alludes to the example itself. Known to be highly effective in promoting peaceful sleep, Box breathing includes giving equivalent time to a nasal breathe in, first breath hold, nasal breathe out, and second breath hold. The rhythm and cadence of box breathing makes it relax. It urges us to concentrate on tallying the corner of each of the four "sides."

Since the in breath and outbreath are equivalent, this method adjusts to your sensory system and help you simply settle and bring your body and mind back to the focus. Box breathing is ideal for relaxing, especially when one of its advantages include promoting-sleep.

Box breathing is an extraordinary procedure for us to deal with everyday stressors as well. The system works in a wide range of stressful circumstances. Hence, it is recommended for everyone. Except children younger than 7-8 years of age, this procedure can be advantageous to anybody, particularly the individuals who need to think or reducing stress.

It is recommended to attempt to rehearse box breathing technique for 10 to 20 minutes on a daily basis, ideally simultaneously of day. On the off chance that that target appears to be unattainable, you may attempt it for a couple of minutes at whatever point you feel and stop it when you become uncomfortable. On the off chance that you practice this technique at list for 5 minutes daily you will see a huge effect in your everyday life.

Locate an agreeable, calm spot to sit or rest

Take your place

Stay calm and relaxed

Take a moment to get comfortable

Don't do anything

Just stay completely relaxed for a few minutes

Make sure there is nothing disturbing you

Notice if there is tension anywhere

If you feel any part tense, release the tension

Adjust your body to release the pressure

Now, close your eyes

1

Inhale through your nose while counting to four gradually

1...2...3...4

Feel the air enter your lungs

2

Hold your breath inside while counting gradually to four

1...2...3...4

Make an effort not to clasp your mouth or nose shut

Basically, abstain from breathing in or breathing out for 4 seconds

3

Start to gradually breathe out for 4 seconds

4...3...2...1

Rehash stages 1 to 3 in any event for 4 minutes, or until calmness returns

1

Inhale through your nose while counting to four gradually

1...2...3...4

Feel the air enter your lungs

2

Hold your breath inside while counting gradually to four

1...2...3...4

Try not to clasp your mouth or nose shut

Basically, abstain from breathing in or breathing out for 4 seconds

3

Start to gradually breathe out for 4 seconds

4...3...2...1

Let's repeat again

1

Inhale through your nose while counting to four gradually

1...2...3...4

Feel the air enter your lungs.

2

Hold your breath inside while counting gradually to four

1...2...3...4

Make an effort not to clasp your mouth or nose shut

Basically, abstain from breathing in or breathing out for 4 seconds

3

Start to gradually breathe out for 4 seconds

4...3...2...1

You are doing great

You are feeling completely relaxed

There is no fear now

There is no anxiety

There is no stress

You can open your eyes now

Or choose to stay in this position for a bit longer

Relish the feeling for as long as you want.

CHAPTER 5: HOW TO CALM EMOTIONS

Regardless of whether it's eating an additional slice of cake, or choosing to go after another job, your emotions influence all that you do. If you are to make every moment count and approach your everyday tasks in a positive manner, you should take care of your emotional health.

Having great emotional health implies you can deal with our emotions, thoughts, and feelings. You can settle on better choices and explore life's difficulties with certainty and versatility. Building your emotional health empowers you to feel content with yourself. You will appreciate important individual connections, and push ahead in life with a sense of purpose and direction.

The impact of emotions on the body

Regardless of whether it's with sweat-soaked palms or an outburst of laughter, your emotions are regularly accompanied by a physical reaction. You have probably experienced a flood of queasiness before accomplishing something nerve-wracking, or a shock of excitement at the possibility of an upcoming occasion.

However, the quick flashes of emotions that you feel in your body are just a little piece of the physical impact of emotions. Your body reacts to your emotional wellbeing from various perspectives — if you are feeling stressed or troubled, you may encounter physical indications, such as insomnia or sleep deprivation, or even hypertension and stomach ulcers.

Poor emotional wellbeing can also affect on your immune system, which is the reason you appear to get more coughs and colds when you are going through a really stressful season or when you are gripped by anxiety, or why you take more time to shake off illnesses when things are strenuous at work.

Also, obviously, when you are feeling somewhat down, you are more averse to taking an interest in the things that advance physical prosperity. When you feel down and out emotionally, or pressured, you are more likely to be tempted to grab an extra glass of wine or to eat unhealthily. Thusly, your emotions influence your basic decision-making skills at the time, which can have an impact on our physical wellbeing.

These physical sicknesses can be a useful sign to you that something isn't exactly great with your emotional health, so you can consider making a move to improve it.

The physical advantages of positive emotions

It's not all awful news. However — there are long haul physical advantages related to emotional prosperity as well, and perhaps the greatest benefit of positive emotional health is the positive effect it can have on your physical health.

For instance, you can likely envision how becoming hopelessly in love prompts feelings of bliss, calmness, and satisfaction; however, did you realize that it's also thought to support the development of new synapses, which improves your memory?

Specific Ways Of Emotions Influence Your Health

Your emotions have an immediate connection with your body that gives them a chance to have a major effect on your psychological as well as on your physical state. With the correct learning, it's conceivable to perceive how ground-breaking your feelings are and how they can assist you with managing your perspective and keeping your body and mind sound.

Have you at any point thought about what you can do to your perspective on life and to the condition of your body with the assistance of the emotions that numerous individuals attempt to stow away? If you consider your emotions when they trouble you, you can help yourself as well as introduce harmony and calmness to your mind.

1. Love

When in love, you may experience a racing heartbeat and your hands getting sweatier. It is brought about by the incitement of adrenaline and norepinephrine, Simultaneously, oxytocin, the "love hormone," makes you feel glad, stable, and minimizes your pain as the "painkiller" zones of the mind are being actuated, and your heart ends up healthier. It is said that wedded individuals live longer than singles because of this.

2. Outrage and anxiety

Outrage is related with disdain, crabbiness, and anger. It can bring you anything from a headache and a sleeping disorder to comprehension issues, skin issues, respiratory failure, or even a stroke. Also, if you're a worrier, outrage can aggravate it even by reinforcing the manifestations of summed up tension issues. So as not to allow your outrage win, step back for a minute, acknowledge why you are irate, and converse with individuals about what's at the forefront of your thoughts. Discover the answer to the issue, and let go of undesirable thought patterns.

3. Depression

Depression is a mental health issue that can lead to emotional distress. This mental state increases your risk of various sicknesses and makes your immune system frail. It additionally causes sleep deprivation in view of a failure to get settled or heaps of hurt thoughts. Depression and being exposed to stress lead to the danger of heart failure. A depressed individual can also experience difficulty with their memory or deciding.

4. Dread

When you are alarmed, the blood truly drains from your face, making you pale. This happens on account of the autonomic nervous system, the fight-or-flight control system. When you face a trigger, veins squeeze off the blood flow to your face and limbs, sending more blood to your muscles and body so you will be prepared for either the flight or the fight.

5. Revulsion

Feeling nauseated by something or, far more atrocious, somebody is one of the most troublesome feelings for anyone to control. Not at all like other emotions such as dread and outrage, which make your pulse accelerate, disgust, or revulsion makes your pulse slow down a bit. You can also feel queasiness or as though something isn't right with your stomach.

This happens in light of the fact that the animosity created by revulsion has a ton of the same physiological components that make up the stomach digestive system. To stay away from this, take a full breath, understand that it's simply your emotions attempting to control your reasoning, and do something contrary to what you're feeling: rather than ridiculing a person or thing, be caring toward them.

6. Shame

In instances of healthy shame, you do not lose your confidence, free-will, and self-esteem. Unhealthy shame generally originates from the past, and, in this sense, unhealthy shame becomes a source of worry. This causes issues, such as overproduction of cortisol, the necessary stress hormone, and this can prompt a heightened pulse and constricted arteries.

To beat shame, quit comparing yourself with others. Figure out how to be sure and unafraid of what individuals say or think. Let them do what they do and say what they want to say. Remember that it's just you who knows reality. Challenge yourself, win the fight, and love yourself.

7. Pride and disdain

Absurd pride originates from adverse thoughts about other individuals together with the belief that there is nobody better than you. This association can make you stressed, which leads to acid reflux, stomachache, hypertension, and so on. The colloquialism "Pride goes before a fall" shows that being proud can prompt an outcome that ends in overlooking potential dangers.

If it's difficult for you to say, "I'm sorry," you need these tips: quit being a perfectionist, and consider your failures as an opportunity for a better attempt. Be progressively compassionate and attempt to comprehend others' emotions. Acknowledge individuals as they may be, document your expressions of remorse, and don't pay attention to shame too much because that is the primary issue that keeps us from being free.

8. Envy

A few people see envy as sweet, however, just when it's not all that much. Normal envy is the thing that an individual feels when they're stressed, or they dread losing a friend or family member. Unhealthy envy can pulverize hearts, connections, and families. The pressure of envy stimulates the pulse and raises blood pressure. You can also have different symptoms that negative emotions bring such poor appetite, huge weight reduction or addition, a sleeping disorder, stomach issues, etc.

In the first place, simply begin to believe your partner, no matter how trite it sounds. Quit comparing yourself with others, and don't mistake fantasy for the real world. These are the best tips for defeating jealousy.

9. Bliss

Bliss or happiness and great wellbeing are connected at the hip, making your heart healthier, your immune system more stable, and your life longer. It additionally causes you to beat stress. As indicated by research conducted in 2015, positive prosperity was found to beneficially affect survival, diminishing the risk of death by 18% in healthy individuals and by 2% in those with illnesses.

Taking Care Of Your Emotional Wellbeing

The flow of wellbeing between the mind and body works both ways, so beyond seeing how our emotions influence our bodies, we can utilize our physical wellbeing to improve our emotional health

Fuel your body with a healthy balanced diet so you can make every second count, and abstain from smoking, and an excessive amount of liquor, which can negatively affect your emotions.

Frequent participation in exercise that you find fun or enjoy will also have various mental advantages — even a brisk 10-minute walk can improve your psychological focus, mood, and energy levels.

Probably most important of all, the act of catering for your body asserts a feeling of self-respect, which is the bedrock of emotional well-being.

Your emotional wellbeing influences how you think, feel, and act, so it's an indispensable part of your general prosperity. Taking care of the emotional side of yourself is fundamental if you are to develop an uplifting point of view, and deal with your emotions, no matter what life tosses at you.

Fortunately, this doesn't need to take a ton of time or exertion — making a couple of little changes to life can help.

Here are a few different ways to calm your emotions:

1. Go through five minutes being mindful

Figuring out how to be increasingly mindful of how you feel at the time can be an incredible method to check out your emotions. Try not to stress if your mind meanders, basically watch the thoughts, and proceed onward. With everyday practice, you'll retrain your perspective to be increasingly mindful.

2. Keep a gratitude journal

Research suggests that recognizing, or recording things that you are thankful for can improve your emotional health. Before you go to bed, write down three things that you are thankful for that day. You'll before long wind up observant of the beneficial things as you go through your daily life.

3. Take a quick walk

Being physically active is an incredible method to improve your state of mind and lessen anxiety. Capitalize on those vitality-boosting endorphins, and get outside for a stroll as regularly as possible, or attempt to discover the closest park or natural area away from the clamor and hectic-ness of the city.

4. Talk with a friend

People are social creatures. Invest energy interacting with friends, or meeting new people, so you have a solid support group of people.

5. Break out of your everyday routine

Doing the same things on a daily basis can be tedious, and leave you feeling dreary. Attempt a deviation from your schedule, regardless of whether it's taking an alternate route to work, or taking up another hobby.

6. Give something

Providing for other people, regardless of whether it's a simple grin, or a couple of hours volunteering, can help your social relationships, and improve your emotional health.

7. Start saying no

Defining limits is an important way to protect your emotional health. Abstain from overextending yourself, and if you have a feeling that you need time to energize without anyone else's presence or input, it's perfectly fine today no to things or ask that they are rescheduled.

8. Start saying yes

Then again, saying yes to great opportunities can be an extraordinary method to open yourself up to new encounters, regardless of whether it is an opportunity to take a shot at something other than what you are used to, or meet new people.

9. Do a digital cleanse

Online networking is great for staying in abreast with what's happening on the planet, yet being stuck to your phones, and seeing other individuals' highlight reels is not always good for your emotional health. Enjoy a reprieve from the social media once in a while, and receive the benefits.

10. Request help

In some cases, we need some assistance to keep our emotional health stable– and that is not something to be embarrassed about. Requesting help when you need it, regardless of whether that is from a friend, a partner or an expert, is one of the most significant things you can do for your emotional health.

How To Clear Negative Emotions

Your emotional health is dynamic, reacting to what's happening around you, your physical health, and many different things. It's alright to have high points and low points — in truth, that is absolutely normal.

Be that as it may, sometimes you will experience negative feelings that do not serve you over the long haul. Also, negative emotions can detrimentally affect your health and wellbeing. So how would you dispose of them?

Below are some different ways to clear yourself of negative emotions, so you can live the life you which to live.

1. Recognize the feeling

When you are feeling blue, do not attempt to escape the feeling, or occupy yourself by relying on unhealthy food, television, or social media. While these might numb the pain for some time, you would not have settled the issue. By recognizing and tolerating negative sentiments, you can begin to get inquisitive about what's causing them, and how you can move forward.

2. Inhale deeply

If you end up feeling furious, or baffled, or unable to sleep because of the thoughts going through your head, take a shot at breathing. Truly, something as basic as taking a couple of full breaths in and out can calm the emotions, and reduce blood pressure.

3. Enjoy a reprieve

Feeling overpowered by the job that needs to be done? Take a break. Regardless of whether you have a deadline weighing down on you, taking a couple of minutes to stroll outside, get some natural air, and gather your thoughts can assist you with coming back with restored vitality.

4. Let it out completely

An extraordinary method to discharge negative feelings is to give them a chance to come all the way out. Relinquish negative vitality with an intense dance session, or a go to the gym. Indeed, even a comfortable walk can help clear the mind.

5. Accomplish something that lights you up

Do you love to paint? Sing? Read? Invest energy with friends? If you discover negative feelings crawling into your life, take a shot at accomplishing something that you can lose all sense of direction in, and you'll before long feel more like the real you.

6. Document your emotions

Journaling can be a brilliant method to process negative thoughts. By taking a couple of minutes every day to write down your thoughts, you can begin to work through your troublesome feelings and take responsibility for your responses to them.

7. Give yourself sympathy

At long last, if life gives you an extreme hand, don't be excessively hard on yourself. Permit yourself to have the full experience of emotions. Notice what has set off the negative emotions; however, don't pass judgment on yourself for having them. Consider what you would say to a friend in a similar circumstance – and be your very own closest friend.

CHAPTER 6: GUIDED MEDITATION TECHNIQUES TO OPEN THE THIRD EYE

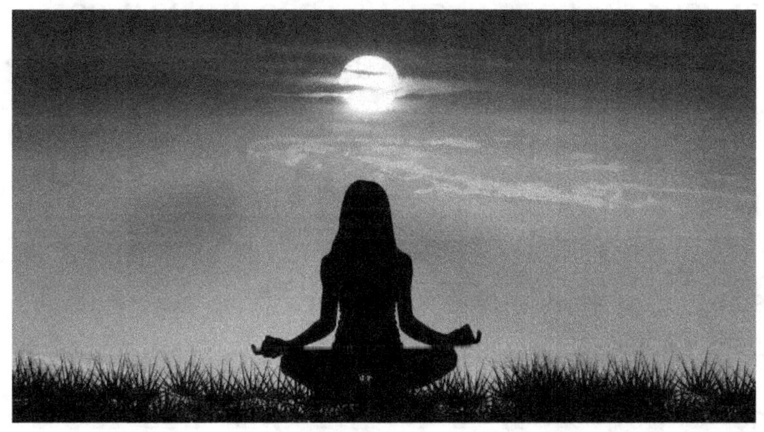

It is the one responsible for the visual abilities which include, seeing visions, flashes as well as symbols. For you to increase the power of the clairvoyance abilities that is in you, you need to apply meditation as one of the vital techniques. Besides meditation, you need to focus on your third eye so that you can trust the experiences that you will have. You have to make sure that the third eye is open if it closed.

In some cases, it may not open immediately, and you have to ask it to open until it does. When it opens, you will feel calm, and warmth runs through your body. The feeling will be as a result of the opening of the body part that was blocked. It has to be awake so that things will run smoothly.

For your closed to open, you need to be preoccupied with a perfect approach to use to open the third eye. It is essential since it functions as an ethereal bridge to connect both the physical and the spiritual worlds. The soul is what makes you a unique and active person, and you have to make sure there is access through the opening of the third eye. It will unlock the higher knowledge, and you will appreciate the experiences you are having from time to time. The third eye does not function on its own but in connection with the hypothalamus gland. That means that it will influence some of your vital biological functions.

Opening your third eye is opening the doorway to the wisdom that is stored in your soul. When you meditate to open your third eye, you will with no doubt have the best spiritual guide. Powerful awakening will happen, and you will appreciate the gift in you that is about to take you to higher levels spiritually. You can choose to go the meditation way so that you can open your third eye. It can be either on your own or with an expert to guide you. When you are doing the guided meditation, the expert will guide you on some steps to make sure that your eye will open. Some of the techniques include and not limited to;

Step 1: Choose a Location

For meditation to hit the primary target, you need to look for a place that there are minimal disturbances. A quiet place is all you need to start with. When you are choosing the site, you need to make sure that you will be consistent. The person to guide you on the meditation should be compatible with you. Your body, as well as the mind, needs to get used to the place that you will choose. A position that you will choose should be in charge of activating your third eye. That too you should consider when choosing the place.

Step 2: Choose the Time with an Intention

After you, through with the first step, work on the second step; that is, selecting the time that you will be going for the guided meditation sessions. You will need to go for the sessions daily so that they can be useful. The time that you will decide to be having the sessions should be reasonable. You should remain fixed at the time that you will choose. Think of the time that will suit you best, and your body, as well as the mind, should be free and in a relaxation mood. You need to avoid scheduling the sessions immediately before or after the time that you take your meals. When you choose a morning, it will work best for you. But that does not mean that any other time is not appropriate. All that is needed when you choose any additional time besides morning is you maintain consistency.

Step 3: Make Some Stretches Before You Begin the Meditation Session

You need to make some stretches before you go to the meeting since you will have to sit longer in the room. You can have a more comfortable time as you meditate on how to open your third eye so that you can realize the power that is in you. When you do this any time before getting into the meditation sessions, you will go to a deeper length of your mental framework. You can try bending over as you try to touch the toes for at least a minute. You can stretch your arms above the head as a way of relaxing. Do not forget to lay on your back and make sure that your feet are in the air at ninety degrees with the body.

Step 4: Position Yourself

Meditation cannot take place while you are standing. You need to adopt a sitting position where you feel relaxed, and you need to cross your legs. If you find this posture disturbing and not comfortable, decide to change and take one which is not difficult for you. A position that will make you relax and focus quickly on your breathing, as well as meditation, is what you need to consider. You should sit on the floor while you close your legs so that you will meditate better on how to open your third eye and access to the hidden spiritual treasures. Your chest should be open and your back straight. Consider placing your hands either on the knees or the lap depending on the position that you will better. Your head needs to be upright and close the eyes gently so that you can get into the world of meditation.

Step 5: Relax

After you adopt a posture that you feel comfortable in, the next logical thing that you need to do is give your body the chance to settle. Meditation cannot take place when you are not relaxed. Be mindful of how your body is feeling and if there are feelings that you need to work on them before the actual meditation, do that. Make sure that your entire body is relaxed and ready to begin the session. Pay attention to all parts of the body each at a time as you sit as well as relax. Shift your mind from any worry that you may be having and be ready to pay attention to the present moment. As you breathe in and out, make sure you are feeling your body expanding and contracting when you take every breath.

Step 6: Breath

Breathing is a crucial technique in meditation. Be focused on how you breathe in and out and put your full attention on how you are breathing. Take deep breaths from time to time on the count of three as you inhale and exhale.

Step 7: Empty the Mind

At this point, you will begin focusing on the third eye, which is at the center of the forehead. With still, your eyes are closed, move your eyes on the direction of the third eye. Throughout the entire meditation process, you need to maintain the focus without moving the eyes from that position. Remaining on the emphasis, count from one hundred moving backwards but do not worry if you are not able to experience the third eye at that moment. You can take quite some time to get used to the process of meditation. It can even take longer to activate your third eye, but that should not worry you. All you need to do is maintain consistency, and with time all things shall work out.

Step 8: Access the Third Eye

When you are through with counting from a hundred backward, it is time that you try to access the sight. Make sure that you had maintained the focus in the previous steps so that this point will be a success. When you have the attention, you will notice that all things are dark apart from your third eye. When the eye is active, your brain will be as well relaxed and functioning on an entirely new level. All the sides of the brain will work in unison, and you will feel the energy that surrounds you. You will feel a new energy level running through your body as well as around you. That is the moment you will know that you got access to your third eye. When you focus on an object or image strongly, that is the time that you know that you are accessing the eye. Your mind needs to be consumed by the object or image fully for that to happen.

Step 9: Work on Experiencing Your Third Eye

Everyone has a different way of reacting to the activation of their third eye. You may experience your mind flashing visual effects and any other experiences and scenes that you may have come through. It can be a way of seeing your thoughts like the way they appear if they can be laid out. As you continue focusing on experiencing your third eye, you will work on opening the eye slowly by slowly.

Step 10: Maintain Your Focus on the Third Eye

You need to remain focused on the third eye for about ten to fifteen minutes. You may have a headache during the very first sessions but know that it is a normal thing that will happen to almost every beginner. There is no need to get worried since the headache will be no more as you get used to the practice. You have to train yourself to fully appreciate your third eye and try to maintain your focus on one image. Amongst the pictures that will appear in your mind, pay attention to one that you decide to choose. Make sure you work to keep the mind centered on the focus that you have made. When you maintain your focus on the third eye, you will find it open slowly. That will mean that you had achieved what your aim was when you were deciding to go meditation. Your third eye will open, and you will have a great experience with the precious gift that is in you.

Step 11: Get out Meditation Slowly

When you finally achieve what you intended, the next thing to do is bring yourself out of the meditation. Remove your focus from your third eye slowly still maintain the relaxation mood that you were in when in the whole process. Your guide will let you know that you have to be aware of your breath. You can choose to count as a way to still focus on your breathing when working on bringing your mind from the meditation.

Open your eyes slowly to end the entire process finally.

In cases when you need to open your third eye any other time, practice the above steps, and it will be easier this time around. That is because it will not be the first time to do that. Work on making your body feel better as well as become in touch with the inner self. However, that will not come immediately, since you need to practice the meditation process, and it will make you go to greater heights. You will be more in touch with yourself as well as the energy in you and around you. That is the main idea of meditating to open your third eye.

There are signs that you will experience to show that your eye is open. Once you manage to open the third eye, you will no longer have self-doubt. You will have a desire to research as well as learn more. You will be more sensitive to spirits, and you may see them from time to time. You will be wiser and will learn from your past mistakes. The chances are that you will be more creative, and you will feel divine inspirations more often. You will achieve great potential, and you will have joy and experience a healthy life once you can connect with the spirits. You will find the world a place of harmony to live in, and you will appreciate your life more. When you finish the self-journey, do not be mean but work to show other buddies with a similar gift with you the way of self-realization.

CHAPTER 7: DEEP SLEEP TECHNIQUES

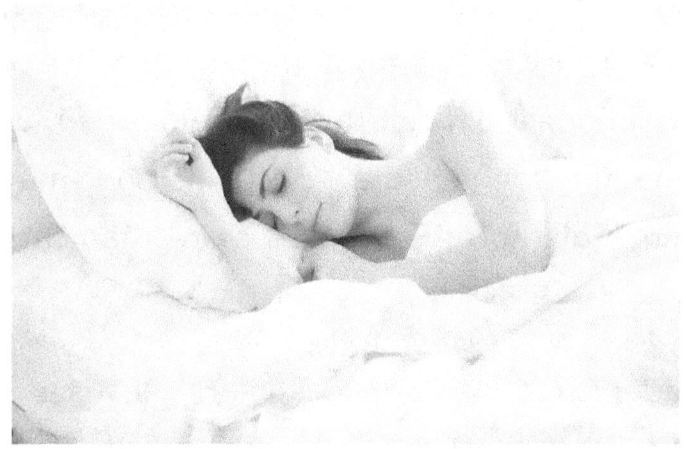

Meditation to Overcome Insomnia

Whether you find it difficult to sleep at night as a result of stress, tiredness, work or several other factors, or you find your sleep unsatisfactory, you might be suffering from insomnia. Insomnia is commonly called difficulty falling asleep, or staying awake, and there two types of insomnia.

Acute insomnia is mostly caused as a result of lifestyle, or circumstances. A security officer on night duty will find it difficult to fall asleep on duty, likewise a first-time dad may find it difficult to fall asleep thinking of his precious wife in labor.

While, chronic insomnia is a complicated type of insomnia. There is no known underlying cause, yet the individual finds it difficult to either fall asleep, or sleep at night for long hours. Such person may also experience disrupted sleep, for more than 3 times a week.

Experiencing insomnia regularly causes mood disturbances, fatigue, stress and difficulty concentrating. Although, insomnia can be caused by factors like anxiety, work related stress, lifestyle, and sicknesses. However, the approach to overcome insomnia is not easy for some persons, yet there is one possible way to overcome not just insomnia but enjoy a long, satisfactory sleep for the rest of your life.

How Does Meditation Cure Insomnia

Meditation is a relaxation technique worth trying, which can help improve your sleep, make you fall asleep easily and also make your sleep satisfactory, such that you wake up feeling refreshed. Meditation harmonizes the mind and body, and also influences the brain and the way it functions. The effect of meditation on your mind and body is that you become calm, and relaxed afterwards.

Effect of Meditation on Insomnia

During meditation, the mind is focused on one thing, which prevents the mind from wandering. Your mind and thoughts are brought to the now moment during meditation. Hence, anxiety disappears and it becomes easier to fall asleep.

During the meditation, your mind and body are been connected to each other, and they both become relaxed and calm, which helps you sleep as soon as you get in bed.

Furthermore, meditation helps boost the hormone called melatonin that regulates the sleep and wake cycle. Without stress, the melatonin level is usually at its peak at night to ensure you get a sound, and restful sleep. However, the presence of stress among other factors that causes insomnia, the melatonin level drastically reduces, thereby insomnia occurs. With meditation, the melatonin level increases because stress has been reduced, and the body is in a relaxed state.

Meditation Techniques for Insomnia

If you want to experience an undisrupted sleep, an intense meditation must be done frequently. There are different techniques of meditating for insomnia and understanding process help us to get started immediately.

• Cognitive shuffling

Cognitive shuffling is a simple meditation technique that can be done alone. It is simply a do-it-yourself technique that shuffles your thoughts to sleep. Here is how cognitive shuffling works, when you lie on your bed, your mind is likely to be filled with different thoughts from your daily activities. You can be worried, and anxious about your bills, relationship, the next day activities, such that you find it difficult to fall asleep. The effect of this shuffling on the brain is it tricks the mind to get into a dreaming state.

Tips to Practice Cognitive Shuffling

- Firstly, getting in bed is important

- Right there on your bed, avoid focusing your concerns. Let your deadline be, the bills, the complicated issue at work. Let it all be.

- Now that your mind is free from your fears and worries, create a new engagement like imagining objects, places, names or movies to meditate on. You can imagine different things, like a teddy bear, a fish, a dog, the sky, the rainbow, or the ocean. Note that, the items you are imagining should not be threatening or scary. For instance, instead of imagining an ocean because you have the fear of water, you can imagine the rainbow or the sky with beautiful stars.

- Ensure your eyes are closed before you begin the cognitive shuffling process.

- Process should be repeated if you are still awake, until you run out of words.

• Sa Ta Na Ma (Mantra)

Sa Ta Na Ma is a powerful meditation technique that works on the brain and its functions to reduce risk of depression and other mental illness. It is a mantra that is usually recited in 3 voices; the singing voice which stands for the action voice.

The whispered voice which stands for your inner voice, and

The silent voice is known as your spirit's voice.

SA TA NA MA chant describes the evolutionary aspect of the universe. Each word in the chant has a meaning.

SA means the beginning.

TA means existence and creativeness

NA means death or the end of life

MA means rebirth

The effect of this mantra is displayed by a balance in emotions, and a settled mind.

Practical steps to Sa Ta Na Ma

- Find a comfortable position. You can sit down or lie down.

- Decide on how many minutes you want to recite the mantra.

- Breathe in and out through your nose and mouth and ensure you sigh after this breathing exercise is heard.

- Close your eyes properly, and place your hands either on your lap, or knee. Make sure your palm is facing up.

- Begin chanting slowly, and press the thumb of your hands, with your four fingers. Count your fingers each starting from the thumb to recite the mantra.

- Keep reciting the chant as a calm and slow pace

During recitation, you have to follow the principles of the mantra.

When you mention SA, you count from your index to your thumb

You count from your middle finger to your thumb when you sing TA

You count from your ring finder to thumb when you recite NA

And final you should count from your pinky finger to the thumb when you mention MA.

- Still in that position, sing SA TA NA MA in a loud voice, your voice should be audible, and ensure you move each of your fingers with each sound. The more you sing, the more you feel relaxed and energetic. However, your soul and spirit should feel relaxed and enjoy the sensation which is moving through your body and mind.

- When you feel relaxed, shift your focus and start singing in a whisper voice. At this point, energy is flowing through the body, waist, and knee.

- Next, be focused on silence. Continue counting your fingers and silently repeat the mantra to yourself.

- After singing the mantra completely, breathe in and breathe out with your arms wide open, and lift the hand above your head. Release your hands down, and exhale again. Repeat process until you feel refreshed or drowsy.

What to Expect When Meditating To Fall Asleep

Your expectations when meditating to fall asleep is most likely to have a sound and deep sleep at night, except you are uncertain about the benefits of meditation. Meditation for sleep is similar to other kind of meditation; however, the approach to each of these meditations is what matters.

When meditating, your meditation technique determines what you will have to do. Albeit, you can start preparing for your meditation exercise, by breathing in and out, lying flat on your back. If you are having a guided meditation, all you need to do is follow the instructions instead of been worried about what to do and what not to do.

Furthermore, all you should when meditating to fall asleep is sleep, but try to avoid any form of distractions.

How to Meditate Before Sleep

There are two ways you can meditate before going to bed, it can be a mindful meditation where you pay more attention to your body and mind, and also having a guided meditation where someone leads you through the process of meditation.

Mindfulness meditation can be done alone, in your own room house and house. While guided meditation is a very easy meditation, it is just for you to follow and listen to instructions from a guide.

Guided Meditation Tips for insomnia

Guided meditation is the form of meditation you engage in with the help of a tutor, or instructor. Ensure that you will not be disturbed, during the course of this meditation.

- Lay down on your back, preferably on your bed or mat. Make sure you are comfortable on whatever you are lying on.

- Close your eyes and prepare your mind for the meditation you are about to engage in.

- Breathe in and out, ensure that your breathing out is audible such that it looks like you breathing out heavily. Make your body feel the heaviness, after which your body will be relaxed.

- Pay more attention to your breathing, and you feel easiness. A natural breathing processes.

- At this point, you will feel your body is relaxed. Feel the way your breath travels through your lungs, and hold your breath. As this is happening, you will begin to feel relaxation in your body.

- You can begin to breathe normally right now, and as you breathe you feel your muscles, joints, and back relaxed.

- Pay more attention to your stomach area right now, where your abdominal muscles are present. Tighten the muscles in your abdomen, and hold your breath for 10 seconds and release your muscles. During this release, feel the difference the tightness of your abdominal muscle and the relaxation of these muscles.

- Repeat the above process 5 times.

- Breathe in and out, tighten your abdomen and release it to relaxation.

Feet

- Divert your attention to your feet, and make them relaxed. The relaxation should be from your toes to your ankles. Tighten your toes and feet, and feel them become heavy and relaxed.

- Focus on your nails, feel them relaxed and let go.

- Pay attention to your thigh area, and feel them relaxed.

- Again, focus on your waist, lower and upper back, joints and feel them relaxed. You will feel the feel heavy, and very relaxed

Upper limbs

- At this point, focus your attention on your arms. Feel them heavy and relaxed.

- Get a sense of how heavy your arm is, and feel the relaxation shift to your elbow, wrist, and fingers become very relaxed.

Face, neck and facial muscles

- Shift your focus to your facial muscles, neck and face.

- Every muscle in your face, your cheeks and chin becomes relaxed, and your entire body is now relaxed.

A deeper meditation for the abdomen

- Locate your center, which is your abdominal region. Imagine there is a bowl on your abdomen. Slowly see the bowl rolling over your abdomen area, and it relaxes every muscle the bowl rolls in contact with.

- The bowl now moves slowly from your abdomen area to your right hip carefully and softly massaging the muscles of the hips it comes in contact to.

- Massaging back and forth all the muscles in your abdomen.

- The ball continues to roll over to your knee, and around your knee. You can feel the tension on your navel melting away. Roll the ball slowly to your toe, and over to your toes, from your small toes to the big toes.

Every part of your body this ball comes in contact with feel the part of your body relaxing.

- Now feel the ball begins to roll upwards away from your toes again. Massaging and reducing tension around your toes, knees, ankles and rolls over to your center, your abdominal area.

- Again, this balls rolls to your left thigh, and your knee, massaging both the back and front of your knee.

With your ball you move this ball to wherever you choose, and how long you want it to be.

- With this ball, massage your knee, and ankle and toes. This ball touches every muscle in your toes, it gently massages them and at this point, you feel your muscle relax.

- Feel the ball roll back up your leg, your knee and thigh muscle and arriving back at your center.

- Shift the focus of the ball to the base of your spinal cord. Allow the ball rest there for 5 seconds, and allow it move up your spine, and near your heart. At this point, you can feel the ball massaging the internal organs in your body. The ball massages the heart, and you feel relaxed.

- The ball rolls to your throat area, and the back of your neck area. You feel your neck area relaxing after the ball massages it. You feel tension reducing around your neck area.

- The ball travels down your arm, and to your wrist. The ball gently massages your wrist, and fingers.

- You feel the ball roll up your arm, to your shoulder and neck. It travels down to your elbow, forearm, and wrist and into the palm of your hands.

- Allow the ball gently massage your palm, and fingers. The ball moves up your arm, shoulder and face and as it reaches up in your face, the ball splits into a hundred tiny balls. You feel them travel around your face, to your eyes, eyebrow, cheeks, chin, teeth, tongue and teeth.

- You feel the ball massaging your face and every part of your face. At this point, you should enjoy this facial massage.

- I want you to imagine as you are lying down the ceiling of your house. Your eyes is still closed, so imagine the ceiling of your room opening itself up, and the roof also opens itself open.

- Still looking at this opening, you will see the beautiful white sky. The sky is clear, bright, and the moon is out and also full, filled with stars. This is a magical peaceful night. You are alone, safe in the beautiful part of your house.

- Watch the twinkling and beautiful little stars, looking down on you and you are enjoying the peace of the night.

- You look again at the stars again, the little ones that are thousands of miles away are not shining so beautiful like the big star closer to you, that is looking at you directly from the sky.

- You are looking deep into galaxy, beyond time, you see a million other stars waiting for you and shining at you.

- Take a deep breath. breathe in a rich air from the infinite and beautiful galaxy filled with stars.

- Feel yourself been a part of these stars, there is no separation between you and them. Feel you are already a part of this wonderful galaxy.

- As you experience this, you become a shooting star, shining across the galaxy like others.

- Slowly you begin to fade into the sky, into the unending space and galaxy.

- You are living in the wonders of this space, where there is neither time, past or future. You feel you are the stars, the moon, and you occupy the pace between the planets.

- You are floating off slowly, as you travel across this universe; you feel your body wants to drift away. You feel peace, wholeness, and love.

- When you are ready, and feel relaxed, you can let go of the galaxy. When you drift off, you will drift into a peaceful and wonderful sleep.

Guided Meditation for Insomnia in Pregnant Women

Meditation for pregnant women can seem difficult; however, the need to be relaxed is very important, to reduce tension, and frustration. Below are some tips to help you meditate as a pregnant woman.

- Pick a comfortable position, you can lie on your back, or sit upright. Ensure you feel comfortable.

- Take a deep breath, and take another deep breath for your baby.

- You are aware of your strong, beautiful and shaped body. You are aware of your baby and how beautiful the baby is.

- Ensure that you feel and observe the sensation that comes as you breathe in and out. As you are breathing in, your body is getting relaxed, and tension is reduced.

- Remember that you are pregnant and meditation can be difficult as this stage; however, take your time to be patient while meditating. Try to avoid every form of distraction around you.

- Find a quiet place to be alone for 10 – 15 minutes. Sit in an upright position, and make sure you are comfortable.

- If you are lying in bed, focus your attention on the bed, by imagining that you are sinking into bed. And if you are sitting, create an imagination of your body in contact with your mattress, and also sinking into it.

- Begin to sense what it feels like to sink into your bed. Notice if you feel lighter, or heavy. Then begin awareness on your body to observe any tension and tightness around your body, from your head to toe.

- Focus your attention on any part of your body you desire, and become aware of the part of the body. Breathe in and out. Get a picture of that part, feel the tension melting away and tightness reducing.

- You can scan your body part 2times in 5 minutes. During this scan, observe and note places that are relaxed or still tight.

- Practice more breathing pattern here. Breathe in and breathe out, for the first 2 minutes, observe your breathing pattern, and focus on your breathing, without a motive to change it. You may start to notice that your breathing becomes slower on its own. You may also notice the way your body moves when you breathe. If your chest rises more than your belly does, it means your breathing is shallow.

- However, a shallow breathing is just a pattern that shows our state of relaxation. If you are relaxed, your belly will rise more than your chest.

- Place your hands on your bell, and feel your baby.

- Observe the movements in your belly with your hands,

- Think about your day, in a structured way. Look back at every activity you did during the day.

Remember when your baby kicked, when you went to see the doctor, when you had a funny and interesting conversation with your friends. Be patient to watch these moments as your brain play them back for you. These flashbacks may seem long or short, it all depends on how your day went. Keep enjoying this flashback, focus your mind on it and avoid been distracted and watch as these events unfold to the present moment.

- Shift your focus back to your baby. Place your attention on your feet, toes and tell them to switch off. You can literally say the word 'switch off' out so that you feel you have told your body parts they are not needed until the next day.

- Repeat exercise and inform your upper limbs, your arms, hands, wrist and fingers to switch off.

- Repeat your breathing exercise again.

- Place your hands on your belly, and say the following words

You are a miracle, and not a trouble.

You will allow me have a restful night

You will be patient with me till I am awake.

You are healthy and strong."

- After saying those words, breathe in and out gain for yourself and your baby.

- Imagine that your baby is falling asleep. Pay more attention on how your baby looks and the way your baby breathes.

- At this point, I believe you should be asleep. If you are not yet asleep, you can repeat exercise and allow your mind get relaxed.

Guided meditation for Insomnia in children

Guided meditation is a type of meditation, where there is an instructor. Little children do not have to that the knowledge to meditate on their own, so their parents can guide them into this meditation using the following.

- Welcome to your happy moment. We will start an adventure right now.

- Make sure you are lying down properly, on your bed, if you feel pain because of the way you lie down, let your parent or guardian know.

- Close your eyes properly and begin to imagine things the sun, how it is so clear and shining. Do not open your eyes.

- Start releasing your body, and everything you are thinking of. So, tighten your muscles, your arms and legs, for a few seconds.

- Let your arms get released, with your legs too. Enjoy the relaxation now, as your muscles are released

- Try the process again, tighten your arms and legs and release them later.

- Start breathing in and breathing out. Make sure you hear the sound that comes out when you breathe in and out.

- Release the air you have breathed in from your lungs, and breathe out.

- Repeat the breathing exercise, breathe in and out and relaxed.

- Now, imagine yourself in a beautiful and dark garden like the wonderland. This wonderland is dark, because it is night.

- You feel the ground is so soft that you feel like sinking into it.

- You feel a gentle and soft breeze on your face and body. The wonderland is so cool and beautiful; you don't want to leave there.

- At this point, you see your body becoming relaxed.

- You look up, and set the beautiful sun set, and the birds flying around in the wonderland.

- You continue walking; you look at the beautiful trees, with fruits on it.

- You keep walking until you see a colorful tent in front of you. The tent is the color of the rainbow. It is so beautiful; you walk into the tent.

- As you go into the tent, you see how beautiful it is. It has a beautiful sofa with the rainbow color, the wall of the tent has the pictures of all your heroes, and you like the way the tent is.

- The tents has different rooms, the living room has a Television set with your favorite cartoon, the kitchen has the pictures of your favorite food, the room has big soft bed, you feel the softness as you touch it, and there is a big pool where you can swim before the kitchen.

- Keep walking around to see how beautiful this tent is.

- Now, you are done looking around this magical tent in your wonderland. You walk out of the tent, and you see another beautiful garden that surrounds the tent.

- This garden is so beautiful. You are walking around and you see a table with two chairs, a jug of juice, and two glass cups.

- You drink a glass of juice, and look around to see if there is anyone around you.

- You then see someone walking towards you; the person is smiling at you. The person is happy, and keeps smiling at you.

- You offer the person a glass of juice, the person receives it happily and drinks.

- You show this person around your magical tent.

- Did you have a beautiful talk with your new friend?

- You hug your visitor softly, and you watch the person go away.

- You breathe in and out and you feel happy and relaxed right now.

- At this point you are feeling sleepy, so you walk back into the tent and walk into your room to lie on your soft and rainbow color bed.

- You tuck yourself into your bed, and place your head on the soft pillow.

- You feel your body sinking into your bed. Your arms are feeling relaxed, and your hips to your toes are feeling relaxed.

- There is a window in your room, so you lie on your side to watch the beautiful dark sky and you also see the big shining star in the center of the sky.

- You smile and feel happy; you tell yourself you are a big shining star.

- You look at the other shining stars; they look beautiful just for you.

- You see them moving together fast; you wonder where they are going. They are going to the galaxy, so you decide to join them.

- You see yourself floating into the dark clouds, and far beyond the clouds, you see more stars.

- You are happy now, and very sleepy.

- You begin to drift away. You are getting sleepier, so you return to your soft bed.

- You cannot open our eyes now, because you are already deep into your sleep.

- You mind and body is now relaxed and quiet.

- At this point, you are fast asleep.

CHAPTER 8: RELAXATION TECHNIQUES FOR ANXIETY

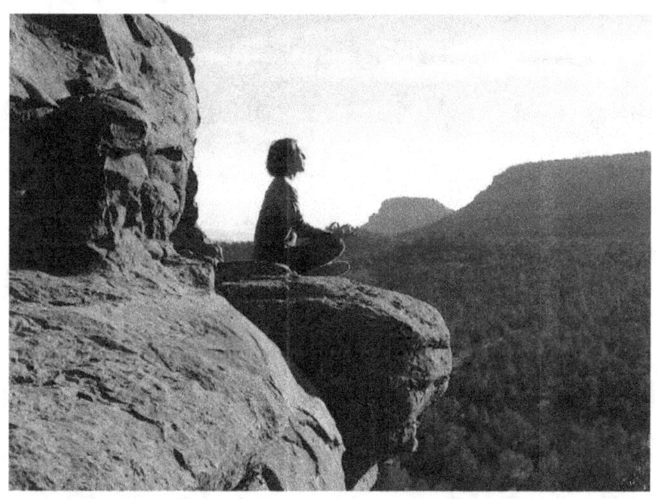

Relaxation is an incredibly effective way of dealing with anxiety, and it applies to all groups of people. It allows the body to activate its natural response to combat stressors. Relaxation comes in many forms and depends on what works best for you. Some of the relaxation techniques that have been proven to beat back anxiety are:

· Relaxation exercises such as muscle relaxation and deep breathing

· Meditation

· Visualization

· Physical activities like yoga

There is a common belief among many people that relaxation involves sitting idle and or doing something you enjoy, like watching a movie or sleeping. No, relaxation is a task that needs concentration and energy input. Its sole purpose is to reduce the effects of stress and anxiety. If your definition of relaxation doesn't meet this goal, then it is far from relaxation. Relaxation achieves this by putting your body to a state of deep rest and restores normalcy such as slowing the heart rate, reducing blood pressure, improve blood circulation, and most importantly checking stress and anxiety. Activities that involve relaxation are those that touch on the most affected organs like the heart, blood vessels, and those in the breathing system. Try things like muscular exercises, meditation, yoga, and deep breathing. Most of these exercises are a form of self-treatment, so you don't need a professional to do them. However, they are quite demanding and require a lot of discipline. If you are the type that needs to be pushed, you might consider looking for a professional therapist to help you do the exercises. The word 'professional' is key because not anybody can make you do things that make you uncomfortable, especially if you're an adult. You need someone that will be hard and a little harsh on you. Also, people have diverse systems that respond differently to changes. If one or two of these exercises don't work for you, look for one that you are comfortable doing and is compatible with your system. You don't have to kill yourself trying to make a particular technique work even you can see that it is not working. Furthermore, all these techniques have been proven to lead to the same results, which is slowing down stress and anxiety. Just don't be too lazy to give a particular technique trial and error period before giving up on it entirely. Remember things take time; you need to give your body a chance to get used to these changes. You will get used to those exercises in no time, and they will become a habit.

There is a thin line between relaxation exercises and meditation exercises. The main difference being that relaxation exercises engage various parts of the physical body while meditation engages the brain. The similarity between them is that they both put the entire body and mind in a state of rest to relief affected parts and organs from stress and anxiety. Both exercises are carried out in systematic steps to the end. Skipping one step will likely jeopardize the whole process. If you are not sure about these steps and the order in which they are done, it is advisable that you seek the help of a therapist who will take you through each step.

There are various exercises that involve relaxation, as discussed below.

Deep Breathing

This is the bedrock of all other relaxation exercises. It is the simplest yet very effective way of keeping your anxiety level in check. It communicates safety to the brain, thus easing tension, stress, and anxiety. It involves improving your breathing by cleansing and opening air cavities for normal breathing to occur. Anybody can do this without any difficulty. It doesn't matter where you do it, anywhere is a perfect place as long as the environment is conducive. Conducive means it is free from noise and particle pollution. There should also be minimal disruption from other people and things. Remember this is a procedure with its own timeline; if you are interrupted say in the third step, you won't resume the exercise from the third step. You will have to start all over again and make sure it goes to completion. This is the procedure:

Identify a quiet spot outdoors, say in the park, or lock yourself up in a clean well-ventilated room. You can also sit down on a chair with your feet touching the ground or lie down with your body straight against the ground or floor. Whatever position makes you feel comfortable.

Sit up straight with your legs straight against the floor or ground, spread them apart or fold them on the knees and let the back of your feet touch. Your back should not lean on anything. Your left hand should be on your abdomen and the right on the chest. Take a deep breathe through your nose for as long as you can, relax the hand on your abdomen to allow the stomach muscles to relax and accommodate more air.

Exhale through your mouth for as long as you can, lightly push your stomach in and contract the muscles to push all the air out.

Repeat this process for like five minutes non-stop. Minimize the movement of the arm on your chest. Focus only on your breathing and try to shut down your brain from all thoughts, whether positive or negative. Make sure the breathing is slow and smooth, don't try to increase the pace. Do this thrice day, each exercise should last at least five minutes, but you can go up to fifteen minutes if you like.

Progressive Muscle Relaxation

This is a two-step process of muscular contraction and relaxation involving various groups of muscles in the body. This exercise is important because it demonstrates how your body physically responds to stress and anxiety. Remember, this is a mental disorder that is not easy to detect, but if we incorporate physical aspects in detection, it will be much easier to know when we are experiencing anxiety. The exercise can be combined with deep breathing to yield maximum results. For you to carry out this exercise, you must be in your best form health-wise; no muscle spasms, no back pains or recent injuries that might put unnecessary strain on the muscles. In case you have or suspect to have any of these problems, consult your doctor before starting the exercise. Here is the procedure.

Put on some comfortable loose clothing or loosen the ones you are wearing by unbuttoning top buttons and sleeves. Remove belts and shoes.

Repeat the steps as those in deep breathe, do it once or twice in this step.

Look at your feet in turn, start with one and spend some seconds looking at it. Move your toes slowly and follow their movement and other induced movements within the foot. Squeeze the muscles as tightly as you can within the foot. Make sure the muscles are tense for some ten seconds before relaxing them. Notice the change and difference between the two exercises.

Repeat this for the other foot and focus on the movement and behavior of the muscles as you squeeze them, and when you relax them.

Notice what tension does to your feet. You can do this by comparing how the foot feels when in tension and when relaxed.

Shift your attention to other groups in your body, such as the hand muscles, stomach muscles, and neck and shoulder muscles. Repeat the process for each and pay attention. Notice the kind feeling associated with tensing various groups of muscles.

Relaxation by Visualizing

This technique involves playing games with the brain by showing it what it desires. It is a very effective technique to combat anxiety because it gives you temporary peace and calmness. You can cultivate this good feeling by repeating this exercise for as many times as possible until it sticks.

If you feel like you're experiencing anxiety, find a quiet place, and make yourself comfortable. You can sit or stand against something like a wall.

Close your eyes, think of your ideal space — a place you would like to be in the real world or just an imaginary one.

Imagine the life there, the feeling, smell of things there, and their sounds. Think about the people you would find in that place and how awesome they are. Let that picture stick in your mind.

Open your eyes and take a deep breathe, severally. Try to feel your mind and notice if you are still experiencing anxiety.

If the anxiety tries to crawl back again, close your eyes once more and retrieve the picture of your ideal place from your mind and go back there. Experience the peace, calmness, and comfort associated with that place for as long as you can.

Repeat this process every time you feel anxious and notice if there are any changes in the completion of the exercise. Remember that the effectiveness of the procedure is determined by the amount of time you give the body to process the change. It never comes that easy, so be patient.

Relaxation through Yoga

Yoga is a workout trend that has taken the world by storm in the last ten years. It combines a series of moving and stationary poses. It also involves meditation, and this makes it an all-round relaxation technique. Apart from increasing stability, stability, and general fitness, yoga is also a powerful weapon to fight anxiety. The following different types of yoga deal with different bodily and mental problems.

Satyananda yoga- this traditional form of yoga is usually considered to be the original yoga. It is centered on meditation though it also incorporates slow poses and deep breathing. This gives it an incredible ability to combat anxiety and other psychological disorders. It is the easiest type of yoga if you are a beginner.

Hatha yoga- this type of yoga involves moderate poses and movements. After mastering all aspects of Satyananda yoga, hatha yoga is the next step to sharpen your yoga skills and improve your ability to keep anxiety at bay.

Power yoga- this is the most intense type of yoga; we can say it is a reserve of the pros. However, this intense pose gives you the ability to deal with intense stress.

Tai chi- most authors don't consider this a type of yoga, but there is a strong reason to classify it as yoga. It involves moving your body in a slow, systematic pattern and accompany it with slow but deep breathing. It is a powerful relaxation method to relieve stress and anxiety.

Like we have seen earlier, meditation is more of a psychological approach to combat anxiety. It involves freeing your mind to choose thoughts with the hope that this will serve as a counter-trigger. There are two main types of meditation.

Mindfulness Meditation

The effectiveness of this method has been put to the test by therapists, physicians, and psychologists for the last two decades. The results have been quite impressive, and it has since been used as a tool to relieve the mind from stress and anxiety. How exactly this method works is still a mystery, but it remains a powerful anxiety therapy method. Some authors have suggested that it works by confining the brain to the present, and by doing that it shuts down traumatic memories and uncertainties of the future. This makes a lot of sense because most stresses are caused by trauma and fear of what might happen. By eliminating these two, the brain can then focus only on current events. Events that deal with reality, free of perceived threats. This is how to practice mindfulness:

Repeat all the steps as with deep breathing above. Focus on your breathe alone, follow every inhalation and exhalation for as long as you can.

Monitor your mind as you focus on your breathing. Try to notice when your thoughts are about to wander and try to follow them. Notice the sounds, smells, and types of worries that your mind picks, then try to bring them back by going back to focusing on your breathing.

Allow your mind to wander once more, not anything particular, but to anything it wants. Let this wandering go on for a while then bring it back again by focusing on your breathing.

Repeat the process for about 10 minutes, twice a day or five times a week. Notice if there is any change in the level of anxiety from when you started the exercise.

Body Scan Meditation

This technique is almost similar to progressive muscle relaxation. The only difference is that it involves listening to the reaction of other parts of the body to muscular movement without judgment. This is the procedure for body scan meditation.

Lie on your back, relax your hands on your sides and keep your legs straight or crossed. Close your eyes and take a deep breathe through the nose and exhale through the mouth. Follow your breathing for like five minutes.

Shift your focus to your feet, contract the muscles of the right foot, and notice the movement of the toes. Feel the effect this tension on the muscles has on different parts of the body as you tense them even tighter.

Repeat this process for the left foot and feel the tension in other regions.

Move to a different body part, say your thighs, and repeat this process. Try noticing the impact this tension has on other parts of the body. Keep moving to your knees, calf, torso, abdomen until you have scanned every part.

After you are done, sit in stillness and quietness and try to remember what you felt in different parts and organs during the exercise.

Repeat this procedure twice or thrice a day and notice the changes in your level of anxiety.

Benefits of Relaxation Techniques

All these techniques have a wide range of benefits both to the body and to the mind. Apart from the benefit of managing anxiety, relaxation techniques are helpful in various other areas as follows:

Improved breathing- techniques that involve deep breathing like meditation and yoga play an important role in opening up air pipes and facilitating the free flow of clean air in and out of the system. Even if one experiences anxiety, chances are that their breathing system will not be harmed.

Mental stability- these exercises and techniques do not only curb anxiety, but they also prevent many other psychological and mental disorders, so you are actually killing two birds with one stone. This is made possible when you keep your mind busy and divert it from the cause of anxiety. This diversion applies to other underlying conditions of the mind.

Spices up one's social life- most of these relaxation activities and techniques are done in groups such as yoga classes and Tai chi. They expose one to different kinds of people and actually make them more sociable. Once someone starts socializing with others, the chances are that they will talk about their problems and get help.

Boosts confidence- anxiety becomes worse if the affected individual considers themselves weak. As soon as these exercises start gaining momentum, you will notice a feeling of self-pride and confidence running through you. This is a hidden benefit of applying these relaxation techniques.

Engages the brain- most people would actually use their free time to worry about ambiguous threats. This will only increase their chances of developing anxiety. Participating in these relaxation exercises will engage the brain, and you won't be thinking about some imaginary threats and problems. By the time you are done with the exercise, it will be time to resume your normal duties, and this keeps your too brain busy to indulge in unhealthy thinking.

Keep in mind that not everyone responds well to anxiety exercises and relaxation techniques. The symptoms may actually worsen for some people. If you notice that these exercises are not doing you any good, go see a doctor immediately for further direction. Seeking professional help is important since you might be suffering from other hidden illnesses.

Explanation of the Reference Technique

This is a technique that attempts to divert the mind from a perceived threat or source of anxiety by shutting down most body reflexes that receive, process, and respond to these threats. It is very effective in offering self-therapy when dealing with anxiety and other psychological disorders. The reference technique follows the following steps.

Find a comfortable and quiet place, and sit down, close your eyes.

Think of things that follow a chronological order like numbers, letters of the alphabet, months, or days.

Start counting from the start to the end. Start counting again but this time in the opposite direction, from the last to the first.

Focus attention on various parts of the body as you do the counting. Notice if there is some reducing tension in some groups of muscles like those in the abdomen, back, and neck. Don't stop counting as you do the listening.

Suspend all muscular activities by turning off the muscles. Don't tense or relax them; just stay still, and focus on your counting.

Release your mind to think about anything, give it the freedom to wander from one thought to another, including your worries. Don't try and stop it if it tries to think about unpleasant things. Just listen and view the pictures without being judgmental.

After allowing your mind to wander on all kinds of thoughts, now start sorting out those thoughts. Removing all negative thoughts, those that you consider unpleasant and makes you worried. Only remain with positive thoughts and statements that make you feel safe and peaceful. Reflect on these positive thoughts for like two minutes.

Open your eyes, take a deep breath, and reflect on the feeling you have just experienced before opening your eyes.

Repeat this for some two times every day and notice whether your level of anxiety is changing from the first day.

Aromatherapy Can Help, Let's use Creativity!

I will compare this unique kind of self-therapy with an expectant woman. Some ladies are known to develop strange behaviors when pregnant. One of them is cravings. You will be surprised to learn some have the weirdest cravings. My first cousin is one such woman. When she was five months pregnant, I happened to have visited her place. Everything was okay until she woke up in the dead of night, demanding petrol. Yes, you heard that, right! She was not using a generator, nor did she have a car that uses petrol. When her husband asked her what she wants petrol for, she gave a hilarious answer that left us in stitches. She just wanted a little to sniff. When we were still treating her demand as a joke, she started behaving weirdly. She looked like she was about to have a panic attack. We had to join the village witches in that ungodly hour with a jar, walking from house to house at 4 AM. We were lucky enough to find a good neighbor who braved the morning cold and siphoned for us some from his car. We gave it to my cousin to sniff, and she became alright, almost instantly.

Aromatherapy works exactly the same way. Aromatherapy is the alternative and integrative medication used in the control of stress and anxiety. The substance used in this procedure is a natural product or products, mostly from plants, to treat anxiety. This technique has been used since long ago for this purpose; it has a commendable record of effectiveness. So why not try it too? This is how the technique is applied to treat anxiety:

· Collect different parts of plants, preferably of the species Matricaria recutita and Lavandula ssp. These plants might not be found in your local area so you might have to buy the whole processed package.

· Extract their oil through simple distillation. Store the oil in a clean container and make it airtight. Store the bottle in a dark space with a temperature of about -20 degrees Celsius.

· Apply the oil to different parts of the body once a day for a period of two to three months. The method of application involves pouring some oil into your palm, rub it on the skin in any body part and spread it slowly and gently with your fingers. Massage yourself slowly for some ten minutes. You can ask someone else, preferably a therapist, to assist in the massaging.

· Repeat this for different parts of the body every day until the two or three months are over.

· Compared your level of anxiety at the end of the treatment and at the beginning to see if there has been any improvement.

The effectiveness of this natural technique in the treatment of anxiety has been proven by medical practitioners the world over. So, why not give it a try? Not as a last option but as a unique approach in combating anxiety. Just like my cousin, maybe you need just one touch of aromatherapy to heal your anxiety.

CHAPTER 9: MEDITATIONS TO REDUCE ANXIETY IN RELATIONSHIPS

Anxiety

You know you are anxious when you feel restless or tensed. Your heart may beat in an accelerated rate and your breathing may quicken. Some people tend to feel tired and weak easily when they are anxious.

It is very important to note and respect the contributions your thoughts make to your anxiety level. Thoughts are the images, memories', beliefs, judgments and reflections that float through your mind and give rise to anxiety. You can ask yourself: "What are the thoughts and images in my mind that keep me feeling as anxious as I feel?"

It is also important to note that fear and anxiety will never solve your problems; instead, they will continue to worsen them. You may unknowingly be substituting practical actions for unnecessary emotions. Meditation breaks down those defenses and excuses. It will help you identify your problems and your resources and help you face your relationship problems head on.

Meditation is a practice with very many benefits. It is a way of training the mind and thought process which will in turn eliminate anxiety. Ellie Shoji, who is an expert in meditation said that the same way physical exercise trains the body, meditation trains the mind.

This practice has more benefits than just helping us have positive thoughts and thinking, it also rejuvenates our physical and mental health. And often when we help ourselves, we help those around us. In this way, solo meditation can positively affect a relationship.

Anxiety can be brought about by a lot of factors. This chapter will focus on anxiety brought about by relationships.

You would agree that relationships can be a very mind-boggling adventure. It is also scary sometimes. Relationships demand full exposure of your true undiluted personalities; this will make you vulnerable to heart breaks and abuse. So, it is normal for one to feel confused and overwhelmed. People generally feel overwhelmed when there are major and scary decisions to be made. For example, it can be scary to have to decide to share a dark secret with a new partner or not. This confusion usually causes anxiety. You can reduce any anxiety your relationship gives you through meditation. Meditation clears your mind and calms it down so you can make major decisions on your relationship effectively.

It is understandable if you feel wary about using meditation to cure your anxiety. You may find it hard to believe that a seated, quiet and isolated activity can help strengthen your social skills, reduce your anxiety level and relationship skills, but research shows it does.

Therefore, let us show you a few ways meditation can prevent anxiety in your relationship.

Strained Communication

Communication is essential for a healthy relationship. If the communication in your relationship is strong, then it has the potential of being healthy and lasting. Strained communication in relationships usually begets anxiety. Meditation can help clear this away. Imagine you are walking in a foggy place. It is difficult to see where you are going but you simply have to keep moving forward. If you panic, it will become more difficult to see through but if you are calm, you will definitely see better. This works in communication too. So much happens in a day and one is usually tired, with a clogged mind. The more you meditate, the calmer you become and the easier it will be to wade through the communication fog and express yourself better.

Meditation will free you from within and any hindrance to your having an effective communication in a relationship, will be easy to deal with.

Toxic Personality

No sane human will want to be found in a relationship with a toxic human. Sometimes, though, the toxicity usually arises as a result of clashes in opposite personalities. You might worry that your personality is causing undue stress on your partner. This worry can cause you a lot of anxiety. You can change your existing scenario with meditation. As a human being, you must have carried your emotional and mental baggage for many years without relieve. Apart from a series of outbursts caused by emotional imbalances, this might even cost you your health. Just like snakes that shed their skin and dogs that shake off water from their fur, you need to shake off the baggage you have carried around before you can successfully rejuvenate yourself. When your mind is free of constant worry, you would find it easy to be happy and, in turn, spread that happiness to others. What you have inside you, is what you would reflect to others around you. This will ease your anxiety and you will find yourself becoming your partners' peace. Your partner will also feel compelled to reciprocate and you would move on in life, a happier and motivated person.

Former Relationship

This is usually a great cause of strained relationships and needless anxiety. Meditation helps you heal from any past heartbreak you might have experienced. During meditation, the mind is content and alert so, it can greatly heal the body, heart and soul. It harmonizes the mind and triggers the healing process.

Gratefulness

A very strong incentive to meditate for a good relationship is its impact on your perspective. Meditation helps you control and regulate your emotions and this power will help you keep a positive perspective. You will find it easier to stay grateful. Gratitude is a very strong indicator of a long-lasting and healthy relationship. Research proves that, over a period of time, you will get used to the things you own and the people that are constantly around you and you will tend to take those things and those people for granted. As a result, you may get to the point where you may focus your energy on the negative attributes of your partner and even forget why you fell in love with them in the first place.

Grateful people are usually more satisfied in their relationships and feel closer to one another. Staying grateful will help you stay focused and appreciative of your partner's good qualities. Your partner, in turn, will feel appreciated, and the bond you share will be strengthened.

Work-Related Stress

You might be going through and experiencing a lot of stress at work. Unfortunately, though, you might bring your stress home to your partner. Inevitably, your partner will get the short end of the stick: a bad temperament, difficult mood swings, lack of affection etc. After a while, this continued pattern will lead to a tensed atmosphere in the home and will widen the gulf between partners.

A research was conducted with veterans returning from war. They were chosen because of the large amount of stress these veterans are known to be under. They used a simple breathing based meditation known as 'sugarcane Kaiya' yoga and their stress and anxiety level dropped drastically. If you can take bold steps in dealing with your stress by using this kind of simple practice, you not only will curb your own stress but also help preserve your relationships with your partners.

It Keeps You Positive

Meditation helps you stay positive, charismatic. It makes you more present, more focused, more productive, and even more creative. Your ability to learn and reason outside the box will improve. It is true that positive emotions help you connect freely with others. It helps us be more open, more approachable and it even solidifies our feelings of connection with other people, even strangers. To explain better: you will realize that on the days you feel anxious and stressed, you are less likely to start up a conversation with the person behind you at a bank. This is because stress makes us selfish and more self-focused. However, though, on the days you feel great, happy and excited, you are more likely to start a conversation or share a joke with a stranger or even notice if someone needs help going through a door. Research shows that laughter, which only occurs when you are feeling positive, makes you more receptive to new persons and helps you create and strengthen relationships. Also, it helps you endure in the face of difficulty. Difficulty can come in the form of a challenging relationship. All of us will face problems in our relationships, but only some of us have natural resilience and an ability to endure and bounce back quickly. Thousands of researches will show that meditation is a strong way to improve happiness and your general well-being. By helping with anxiety and even depression, it can help keep you in a positive frame of mind that has enormous benefits.

Your Connection

As noted earlier, after a while partners tend to feel disconnected from each other. In a research conducted on loving-kindness and compassion based on meditations, it was realized that these types of meditations can greatly help partners feel more empathetic and connected. Meditation can help train and help you to feel more compassionate and loving. Other research shows that empathy and compassion contribute a lot, positively, to your health, well-being and happiness: improved happiness, decreased anxiety and depression, and even a longer life not to mention stronger and healthier relationships with other persons.

To further convince you of the effectiveness of Meditation, let us consider Research Works carried out on Meditation and Generalized Anxiety Disorder

This research was to prove the benefits of meditation on generalized anxiety disorder and the results have been positive. In 2013, a random yet regulated test was carried out with ninety-three persons that had been diagnosed with GAD. These persons had to go through eight weeks of manualized Mindfulness-Based Stress Reduction in a group program and also an Attention Control or Stress Management Education.

After the test, it was obvious that MBSR had helped with significantly larger reductions in anxiety for three out of the four study forms. These persons also showed a more profound increase in positive self-motivating statements.

Easy Steps to Help You Overcome Anxiety in your Relationship

1. Be Calm

You must have found yourself criticizing everything you do. It is normal, we all have an inner critic in us that thrives in cooking up doubt and filling our minds with anxious thoughts. If this occurs, the very first thing you should strive to do is calm yourself so it doesn't spiral out of control. Meditation calms the nervous system and gives you an opportunity to create separation between you and those negative thought lines. You will come to realize that you do not have to react to every thought that flips into your mind. So, take in some long calming breaths and put aside some good meditation time.

2. Process the Facts

The next step is to figure out the exact negative situation that is making you anxious. This is because, most of the things that make us anxious, are based on thoughts we make up in our own head. So if for any reason, your relationship is causing you anxiety, search yourself and find out why it is and while doing that focus only on facts not opinions. This will help you fully understand your present situation rather than some imagined failure.

3. Self-Care

When you begin to feel anxious about your relationships, it is necessary to concentrate on taking good care of yourself. Instead of acting out against your partner or trying to get reassurance, do only those things that will promote your wellbeing and make you feel confident.

4. Heal from Within

You would have noticed by now that these steps are all the necessary steps you need to take to gain control over yourself and definitely not your partner. Heal yourself from within, this is really the only way you can cope with these potentially harmful feelings, because they come from within. It is possible to worry and be aware of yourself without being anxious.

5. Mindfulness-Based Meditation

Meditation used to effectively treat anxiety disorders usually comes in the form of Mindfulness-Based Meditation. This form of meditation can be dutifully traced to the mindfulness movement started by Jon Kabat-Zinn who is the founder of the Mindfulness-Based Stress Reduction Approach. The simple aim of the Mindfulness-Based Stress Reduction Approach is to learn to completely avoid troubling thoughts. You can achieve this by practicing awareness, figuring out the cause of anxiety in your body, knowing your thought process and learning how best to do away with your painful emotions.

MBSR works better when practiced with an instructor, but you can achieve the same result from courses available online.

Steps for Mindfulness Meditation to Distill Relationship Anxiety

Below are easy steps to follow to get started today:

1). Sit upright in a chair with the palms of your feet flat on the floor.

2). Focus on your breath. Pay attention to your breathing. Do not try to vary how you are breathing, just watch and observe your body as you breathe in and out.

3). You might get distracted or find that you want to focus on something else. Ignore and defiantly resist this longing and continue to concentrate on your breathing.

4). Anxious thoughts may at this point, cross your mind. It is expected. Do not shut them down rather, acknowledge them and then calmly go back to awareness of your breathing.

5). Keep up with this calm, non-critiqued observation for close to ten minutes.

6). Slowly open your eyes and take note of how you feel. Don not try to analyse the feeling, just observe.

It is easy to practice meditation. All you have to do is accept the world, the environment around you. Be curious. Observe. This meditative practice, after a while, will spill into other parts of your life, as you concentrate on yourself observing rather than focusing on anxious and difficult situations and over-reacting.

Difficulties in This Meditation

There are several detractors to meditations. You might find that it is hard to meditate or be mindful. You might find it difficult to concentrate without letting the critique voice speak or you may feel too busy or restless as though there is simply too much to do, to be lounging around, breathing in and out. People are wired differently. Some people simply find it difficult to just do nothing. They are constantly on the move and they are used to it. Also, sometimes, you might realize that you cannot prevent the difficult thoughts from taking over even when you try to relax.

The best advice that will help to overcome these obstacles comes in two ways:

Respect the process

You should understand and recognize that this will take some time. You will not become an expert at this in a day. When you first start meditating, you will feel strange. Your mind will bug you, make you feel that you are wasting your time, just sitting around there doing nothing literal. You will get even get angry and fed up. Even with all this, though, religiously continue with it. It will definitely get better. Do not expect your very first meditation practice to be easy at all, it may not. Funny as it sounds, it does take practice to master the art of doing absolutely nothing. In the end, it will become easier.

Create time

Since you have identified the fact that the Meditation will take time, it is best to make out time for it. Put in a time for it on your schedule just like you put in a job or an appointment. Do not make it an option not to practice. There is no reason why practice should be skipped for a day. Just discipline yourself. Tell yourself that you need to get it done. Most times, when you find that you have got a lot of things to do and achieve and you still try to fit in time for a calm moment, you will discover, later, that that calm moment helped you to go back to your day more aware and faster at solving problems.

Update a diary with records on your growth and truthfully indicate if your anxiety is reducing. After a short while of constant meditation, you should ask yourself questions like: When anxious thoughts flashed through your mind, were you able to examine them without criticizing or judging them? Did you succeed in acquiring a moment of focused observation? Did you feel calm, relaxed and aware? If after a while, you are still plagued with troubling thoughts and anxiety that is repetitive and harsh, go ahead and have a talk with your doctor about other treatment options.

How to Practice Meditation for GAD

If you are suffering from Generalized Anxiety, mentioned earlier, performing constant daily meditation can assist you in overcoming anxiety and in reducing increased tension in your body. Yoga has a lot to do with meditation so If you have ever taken a yoga class, you have taken a good first step and you are already on the right path to achieving the peace you seek.

Again, at first, you will not need a whole lot of time to meditate. A few minutes may be a you need. Make efforts to make out a few minutes each day to meditate. As you become more and more familiar with the process, and as you figure out how to relax and discover what it feels like to be calm, you can slowly increase that time.

GAD is simply unrelenting worry, worry that would not go away. Meditation helps you to learn to live with those worries and thoughts without giving them the power to upset you. When you finally achieve that, your distress is more likely to reduce.

CONCLUSION

Even though anxiety can be difficult to manage, people should not feel like they have to struggle with it forever. The first step to recovery is often acknowledging its many symptoms such as sweating, trembling, a racing heart, and nervousness. Making efforts not to let anxious thoughts control your day and decisions can be difficult, but it can help to keep you from having panic attacks. Learning how to ride out the symptoms of anxiety and panic takes a lot of practice and it is important not to get discouraged or start avoiding situations due to anxiety.

Sometimes dealing with anxiety can be too much for someone to handle without professional help. It can be difficult to admit what seems like defeat and call a doctor, but it can be the best way for people with severe symptoms to find relief. There is a wide array of options to choose from when picking a doctor. If a person is too overwhelmed by their choices, they can always go to their primary care doctor who can then refer them to a trusted psychologist or counselor.

After establishing a relationship with the therapist, you can then work on establishing trust and working toward a long-term goal with milestones along the way.

It's perfectly astute and correct to assume that this moment within your life may be all that you have. Thus, learn to embrace it and stop feeling bogged down by other people's judgment of you. If you made mistakes in the past, don't make them in this moment and don't waste this moment by letting your thoughts drag you into the past. If you can make things right with people by apologizing, do so. If you can't, learn from the mistake and don't make it again.

Anxiety can go away, but you have to understand that a thought that you have today isn't' important in the overall picture of life. If you waste this moment on negative thoughts, you go into the next moment with negativity already there in your life. If you fill this moment with a positive action, you reinforce your value and you move forward into the next moment as a better person than you were a moment ago. Thus, it follows that building up your confidence should be done moment by moment. I made a friend a cup of coffee because I knew that she was lonely. It made her feel better. It made me feel better. Small gestures that take selfish thought out of the picture help to build up positivity that helps to pull you out of the pits of depression. I helped a lady with her shopping because she was older and struggling. When you give, give with no expectations of return because that's the kind of giving that helps you to build up your confidence in yourself. You do things because you know they are positive things to do. You don't do them for thanks or for something given in return. When you incorporate giving into your everyday life, it's a positive reminder to yourself that you have value.

Even after a great loss in your life, you need to feel that value explained above. You may lose your purpose for a while, but if you make this your aim in life, you begin to feel you are building strong roots that will take you through all the pitfalls of life with your head held high, knowing that your personal strength and roots will help you through the bad times that come into your life. Anxiety is a phase. It's a stopping point to reassess who you are and make yourself even stronger and more confident, taking you back up the path to happiness.